Hair Pathology
with Trichoscopic Correlations

Hair Pathology
with Trichoscopic Correlations

Mariya Miteva, MD

Associate Professor
Dr. Phillip Frost Department of Dermatology and Cutaneous Surgery
University of Miami Miller School of Medicine
Miami, Florida, USA

CRC Press
Taylor & Francis Group
Boca Raton London New York

CRC Press is an imprint of the
Taylor & Francis Group, an **informa** business

First edition published 2022
by CRC Press
6000 Broken Sound Parkway NW, Suite 300, Boca Raton, FL 33487-2742

and by CRC Press
2 Park Square, Milton Park, Abingdon, Oxon, OX14 4RN

© 2022 Taylor & Francis Group, LLC

CRC Press is an imprint of Taylor & Francis Group, LLC

Library of Congress Cataloging-in-Publication Data

Names: Miteva, Mariya I., author.
Title: Hair pathology with trichoscopic correlations / by Mariya Miteva.
Description: First edition. | Boca Raton : CRC Press, 2022. | Includes bibliographical references and index. | Summary: "This highly illustrated text will help clinicians become familiar with how to obtain an optimal specimen and how to understand the pathology report, in order to create an individualized approach in management"–Provided by publisher.
Identifiers: LCCN 2021011777 (print) | LCCN 2021011778 (ebook) | ISBN 9781138313538 (hardback) | ISBN 9781032049199 (paperback) | ISBN 9780429457609 (ebook)
Subjects: MESH: Hair Diseases–diagnostic imaging | Dermoscopy–methods | Hair–diagnostic imaging | Hair–pathology | Scalp–diagnositc imaging | Scalp–pathology
Classification: LCC RL151 (print) | LCC RL151 (ebook) | NLM WR 450 | DDC 616.5/46–dc23
LC record available at https://lccn.loc.gov/2021011777
LC ebook record available at https://lccn.loc.gov/2021011778

ISBN: 978-1-138-31353-8 (hbk)
ISBN: 978-1-032-04919-9 (pbk)
ISBN: 978-0-429-45760-9 (ebk)

Typeset in Times LT Std
by KnowledgeWorks Global Ltd.

Contents

Preface

The objective of this text is to demonstrate the power of the trichoscopic-pathologic correlation for the optimal management of hair disorders. Clinicians will become familiar with to obtain the optimal specimen and how to understand the pathology report in order to create an individualized approach in management. Pathologists will become familiar with the trichoscopic morphologic correlation of hair disorders, with diagnostic clues and the most common pitfalls in hair pathology.

Special acknowledgements to my dear friend Giselle Martins, MD, for her invaluable support with sharing many clinical and trichoscopic images from her practice and to Aisleen Diaz, MD, for her outstanding work on collecting and organizing the trichoscopic images. All other contributions are acknowledged in the book.

Mariya Miteva

Contributors

Giselle Martins MD
Hair Department
Dermatology
Santa Casa de Misericórdia de Porto Alegre
Brazil

Rui Oliveira Soares, MD
Tricology Coordinator
Cuf Descobertas Hospital
Lisbon, Portugal

Hair and Scalp Dermoscopy (Trichoscopy)

1

An Introduction

Contents

GENERAL CONCEPTS

Trichoscopy is a type of an epiluminescence microscopy (ELM) utilized to visualize the skin's undersurface and the hair shafts on the scalp. Any type of dermatoscope can be used for trichoscopy including handheld (pocket) dermatoscopes and videodermatoscopes. Since trichoscopy aims at analyzing simultaneously many hair shafts in a single field of view and most hand-held dermatoscope lenses measure less than 30×10 mm, it is most practical to attach a hand-held dermatoscope to a smartphone/iPad or to a digital camera to expand the overview on a screen. Available options include Handyscope (FotoFinder systems, Bad Birnbach, Germany), DermScope (Canfield, Fairfield, NJ), and most of the DermLite dermatoscopes (3Gen Inc., San Juan Capistrano, CA). Hand-held dermatoscopes provide magnification of 10×, whereas videodermatoscopes provide a variable magnification from 10× to 140× and have photo-storage software applications allowing for real-time comparing of "before" and "after" pictures. There are also portable USB dermatoscopes that offer alternative to video-dermatoscopes (FotoFinder leviacam, 20–70×, 13 megapixels). Currently, most published trichoscopy data has been obtained with the FotoFinder videodermatoscope.

MAIN USE

1. Suspect scarring from non-scarring alopecia (Figure 1.1)

2. Select the optimal site for a scalp biopsy (dermoscopy guided scalp biopsies) (Figure 1.2)
3. Monitor progress on treatment
4. Guide the treatment approach (for example, broken hairs and exclamation hairs are markers of active disease in alopecia areata)
5. Diagnose hair shaft disorders *in vivo* and *ex vivo* on plucked or pulled hair samples (Figure 1.3)

SPECIFICS

1. Alcohol solution, gel or water is used as immersion fluid to reduce the glare from the stratum corneum by eliminating the air interface and allowing for increased light penetration into the skin.
2. Dry trichoscopy (without immersion fluid) is utilized to study scaly and keratotic scalp conditions as well as foreign materials such as debris from leave-in hair products and medications, hair dye particles and camouflage fibers; each trichoscopic exam should start with dry trichoscopy (Figure 1.4).
3. Polarized light cancels the reflection from the stratum corneum and thus most light is reflected from the deeper layers of the skin, particularly from the vasculature and the collagen.
4. *Non-polarized contact dermoscopy using immersion fluid* is the standard technique for trichoscopy.
5. Vessels are studied better with non-contact polarized dermoscopy at higher magnifications (40× and

Lost follicular openings

Small tufts with peripilar casts

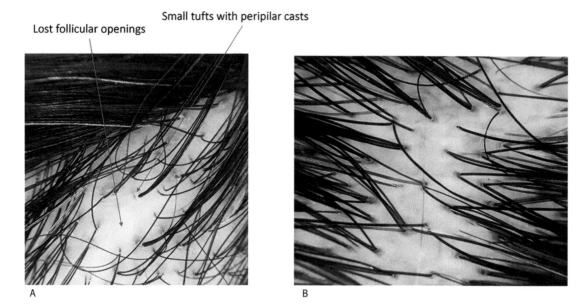

A   B

FIGURE 1.1   Two patients with thick hair density. (A) is suspicious for scarring alopecia based on the trichoscopic findings of lost follicular openings and small tufts of hairs surrounded by peripilar casts. (B) shows preserved follicular openings and is from a patient with non-scarring alopecia (telogen effluvium) (×10).

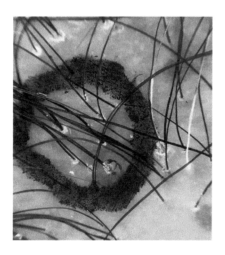

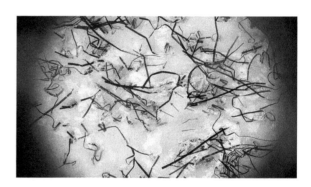

FIGURE 1.3   Trichoclasis (clean transverse hair fracture) in a young man with trichoteiromania – trichoscopy allows making the diagnosis by recognizing the numerous fracture sites where the cuticle is missing (×20).

FIGURE 1.2   Dermoscopy helps to select the optimal site for the biopsy as in this case of lichen planopilaris, which shows peripilar casts around the proximal emergences of the hair shafts (×10).

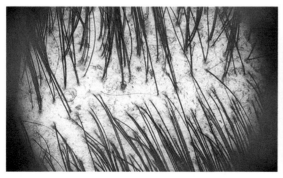

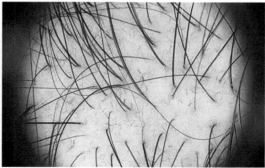

FIGURE 1.4   Dry trichoscopy shows synthetic pigment and fibers used by the patients to camouflage the area of thinning (androgenetic alopecia; ×20).

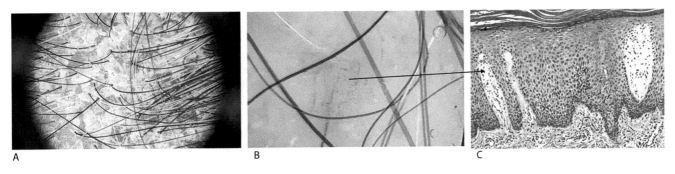

A   B   C

FIGURE 1.5   (A) Dry trichoscopy in psoriasis demonstrates thick white interfollicular scales (×20). (B) After using immersion solution to hydrate the scale, lace-like vessels (with serpentine shape and open end) are noted (×70). (C) These vessels correspond to the elongated and dilated capillaries in the dermal papillae on pathology.

up); if there is a thick scale obscuring the vascular pattern as in psoriasis, immersion fluid should be used to hydrate the scales first (Figure 1.5).

PEARLS

1. The trichoscopic exam in non-scarring alopecia includes parting the hair in the midline and obtaining several images along the midline ranging from 20× to 50× for each site. This allows the assessment of the hair shaft variability and vascular pattern.
2. In men with male pattern hair loss, additional images should be obtained from the occipital scalp (as a reference for normal hair density), the bitemporal scalp and the vertex.
3. In patchy alopecia, the exam should start with assessing the center of the patch for presence of follicular openings (non-scarring alopecia) vs. their absence (scarring alopecia).
4. Dry trichoscopy should be used if there is suspicion of scarring alopecia as the immersion fluid hydrates the peripilar scales (casts) and they disappear.
5. Hand-held dermatoscopes visualize the peripilar casts clearer compared to videodermatoscopes (personal observation).
6. The frontal hairline, the sideburns and the eyebrows should be evaluated in every woman as part of the hair exam given the rising prevalence of frontal fibrosing alopecia; loss of vellus hairs in the frontal line is a clue to early disease.
7. Most common morphologic structures and patterns at summarized in Table 1.1.

TABLE 1.1   Most common morphologic structures and patterns (Figures 1.6–1.24)

STRUCTURES	DEFINITION	TYPES	CLINICAL DIAGNOSES
Dots	– Small clinically non-visible round to polycyclic structures – Usually associated with follicular openings (isolated from follicular openings in nevus sebaceus)	*Yellow dots*: yellow to pink concentric structures devoid of hairs or associated with vellus hairs, cadaverized hairs or black dots; represent dilated infundibula plugged with sebum and keratin; not visible in skin types IV –VI; not visible in prepubertal children	– Alopecia areata – Alopecia areata incognito – Androgenetic alopecia (irregular distribution; mostly in frontal scalp) – Discoid lupus erythematosus (polygonal yellow dots and yellow dots with a red spider) – Dissecting cellulitis of the scalp (3D yellow dots)
		Black dots (cadaverized hairs): amorphous residue of broken hairs at the surface level – fracture occurs prior to exiting the scalp; visible only in patients with dark hair	– Alopecia areata (correlate with disease activity) – Trichotillomania – Tinea capitis – Pressure induced alopecia – Syphilitic alopecia – Central centrifugal cicatricial alopecia

(Continued)

TABLE 1.1   Most common morphologic structures and patterns (Continued)

STRUCTURES	DEFINITION	TYPES	CLINICAL DIAGNOSES
		Brown dots: monomorphous brown concentric structures marking the empty follicular ostia	Anthralin stained follicular ostia in alopecia areata
		Red dots: erythematous, polygonal or concentric structures; correspond to perifollicular inflammatory infiltrate with red blood cell extravasation	Discoid lupus erythematosus (specific)
		Pinpoint white dots: 0.2–0.3 mm regularly distributed white circular structures ("starry sky pattern"); correspond to the acrosyringeal and follicular ostia	– Normal scalp in skin types IV-VI (regular distribution) – Scarring alopecia in skin types IV-VI (irregular distribution)
		White dots: white circular structures larger than 0.3 mm; they correspond to: (a) fibrotic tracts replacing preexisting follicles or (b) empty follicular ostia in skin types IV-VI	– Scarring alopecia (mostly lichen planopilaris, at the margin of the patch) – Alopecia areata (skin types IV-VI)
		Dirty dots: interfollicular brown, yellow or black clumps of less than 0.1 to 0.5 mm; particulate debris of exogenous sources	Normal scalp of prepubertal children and elderly patients
Broken hairs	Hair shafts of variable shorter length with broken distal end and abnormal structure; result from internal (alopecia areata, tinea capitis, syphilitic alopecia) or external damage (trichotillomania, chemotherapy induced alopecia) that leads to fragility and fracture of the hair shaft after exiting the scalp	*Exclamation hair:* thicker distal end and proximal narrowing	Alopecia areata
		Comma hair and corkscrew hair: bent or twisted structure	Tinea capitis (specific)
		Flame hair, tulip hair, hair powder, V-sign: various shape and structure as indicated by their given names	Trichotillomania (flame hairs also in alopecia areata, chemotherapy induced alopecia, radiotherapy induced alopecia, central centrifugal cicatricial alopecia)
		Coiled hair: irregular shape and a jagged end (resembles a question mark)	Trichotillomania
		Broom hairs (trichoptilosis): short hairs with split ends emerging from the same ostium	Lichen simplex chronicus
Regrowing hairs	Individual short hair shafts that emerge in the process of hair regrowth	*Upright regrowing hairs:* normal thickness (thicker than 0.03mm), pigmented and tapered distal ends	– Telogen effluvium – Alopecia areata incognito – Alopecia areata
		Circle hairs (pigtail hairs): Short regrowing hairs of uniform thickness (thinner than 0.03mm), color and coiled shape	– Alopecia areata – Chemotherapy induced alopecia

(Continued)

STRUCTURES	DEFINITION	TYPES	CLINICAL DIAGNOSES
Peripilar casts	Layers of tightly attached scales surrounding the emerging portion of one or more hair shafts	*White flat/tubular* perifollicular scaling	– Lichen planopilaris – Discoid lupus erythematosus – Frontal fibrosing alopecia
		Yellow "starburst" scaling surrounding tufts	Folliculitis decalvans
Peripilar halo	Concentric annular discolorations surrounding the emerging portion of a hair shaft	*White/gray halo* – corresponds to perifollicular fibrosis at the infundibulum	Central centrifugal cicatricial alopecia
		Salmon colored halo – corresponds to amyloid deposition in perifollicular distribution	Amyloidosis of the scalp
Peripilar sign	Brown annular discoloration surrounding the hairs at the emergence on the scalp; corresponds to mild lymphocytic infiltrate and fibroplasia at the infundibulum		Androgenetic alopecia
Keratotic plugs	Keratotic masses plugging the follicular ostia		– Discoid lupus erythematosus – Dissecting cellulitis of the scalp
Hair tufts	More than 6 hairs emerging from the same ostium	– Small tufts (less than 4 hair shafts)	Lichen planopilaris Discoid lupus erythematosus
		– Tufts (more than 6 hair shafts)	Folliculitis decalvans
Vascular structures	Vessels of different shape and morphology observed with polarized non-contact trichoscopy at higher magnification (x40 and more) form different patterns; they correspond to telangiectasia	Simple red loops Arborizing vessels (thin)	Normal scalp
		Arborizing vessels (thick)	Discoid lupus erythematosus
		Twisted red loops (glomerular like vessels) Lace-like vessels	Psoriasis
		Numerous giant capillaries	Dermatomyosistis
		Hairpin, serpentine and comma vessels	Seborrheic dermatitis

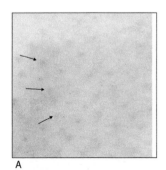
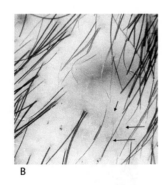

FIGURE 1.6 (A) Yellow dots in alopecia areata and (B) 3D-yellow dots in dissecting cellulitis of the scalp (×10).

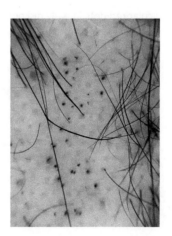

FIGURE 1.7 Black dots (cadaverized hairs) in alopecia areata (×10).

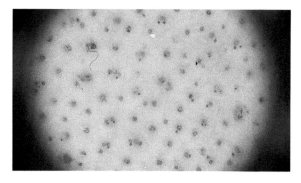

FIGURE 1.8 Brown dots in alopecia areata correspond to anthralin deposited in the follicular ostia (×20).

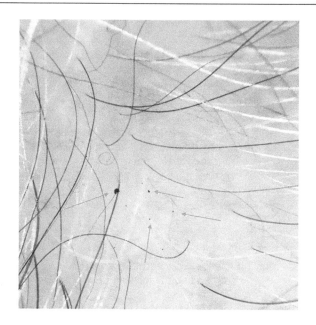

FIGURE 1.11 Dirty dots in an elderly patient (×10).

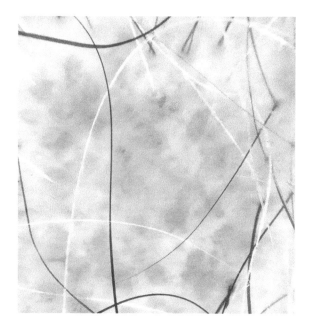

FIGURE 1.9 Follicular red dots in early discoid lupus erythematosus (×10).

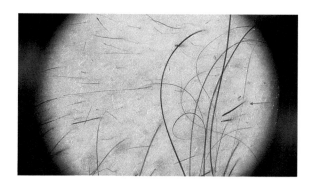

FIGURE 1.12 Exclamation hair in alopecia areata (×20).

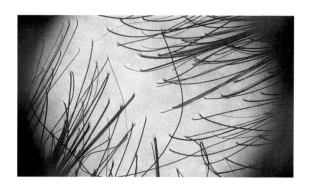

FIGURE 1.10 Pinpoint dots in a patient with skin type IV (×20).

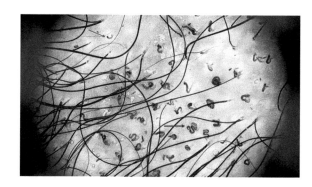

FIGURE 1.13 Comma hairs (red) and corkscrew hairs (blue) in tinea capitis (×20).

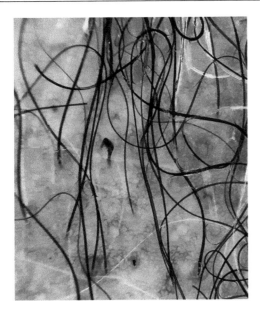

FIGURE 1.14 Coiled hair and cadaverized hair in trichotillomania (×10).

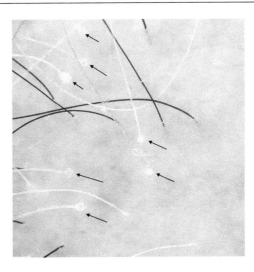

FIGURE 1.17 Peripilar white casts in frontal fibrosing alopecia (×10).

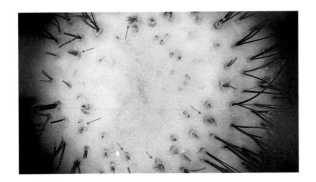

FIGURE 1.15 Broom-like hairs in a case of lichen simplex chronicus (×20).

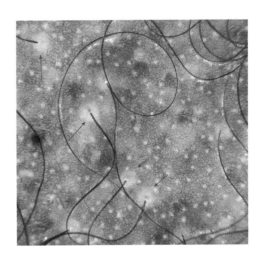

FIGURE 1.18 Peripilar white/gray halo in central centrifugal cicatricial alopecia (CCCA). Note also the pinpoint white dots in background (×10).

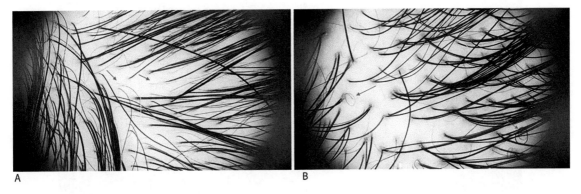

FIGURE 1.16 (A) Upright regrowing hairs (red) after treatment with minoxidil and (B) circle/pigtail hairs (blue) in a patient with androgenetic alopecia (x20).

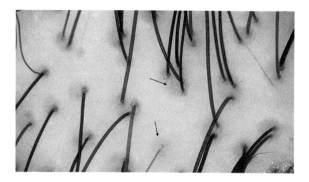

FIGURE 1.19 Peripilar sign in androgenetic alopecia (×40).

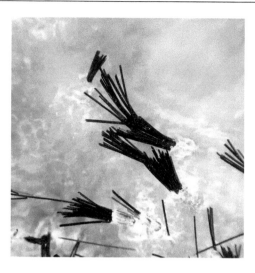

FIGURE 1.21 Tufts (more than 6 hairs exiting from the same follicular ostium) in folliculitis decalvans (×10).

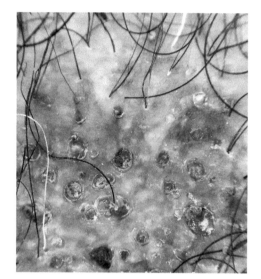

FIGURE 1.20 Keratotic plugs in discoid lupus erythematosus (×10).

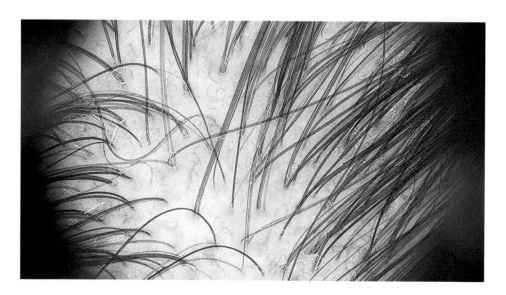

FIGURE 1.22 These arborizing vessels are normal finding of the posterior scalp in men (×20).

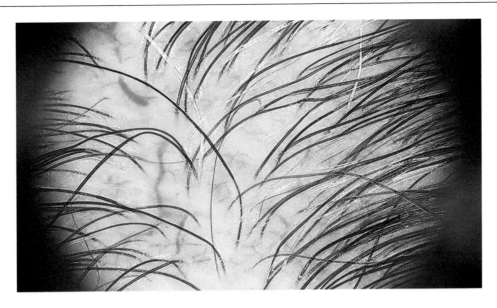

FIGURE 1.23 Thick arborizing vessels in connective tissue disease (×20).

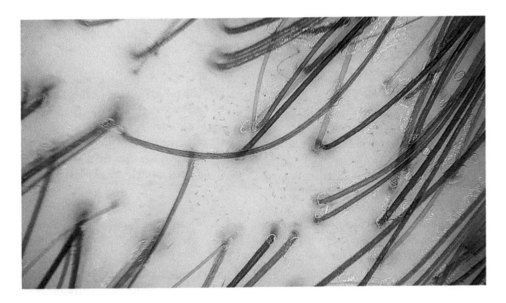

FIGURE 1.24 Simple loops in normal scalp (×50).

FURTHER READING

Miteva M, Tosti A. Hair and scalp dermatoscopy. J Am Acad Dermatol. 2012 Nov;67(5):1040–8. doi: 10.1016/j.jaad.2012.02.013. Epub 2012 Mar 8. Review.

Pirmez R, Tosti A. Hair and Scalp Dermatoscopy (Trichoscopy). In Miteva M, ed. *Alopecia*. 1st ed. Elsevier; 2018: 43–57.

Rudnicka, L, Oszewska M, Rakowska A, eds. *Atlas of Trichoscopy – Dermoscopy in Hair and Scalp Disease*. 1st ed. London: Springer-Verlag; 2012:11–46.

Vincenzi C, Tosti A. Trichoscopy patterns. In: Tosti A, ed. *Dermoscopy of the Hair and Nails*. 2nd ed. Boca Raton: CRC Press; 2016:1–20.

Normal Scalp and Hair on Trichoscopy

2

Contents

FOLLICULAR OSTIA

Original studies on trichoscopy of the normal scalp are limited and include only Caucasians.

The normal follicular ostia/follicular openings mark the sites of the proximal emergence of the hair shafts from the scalp. The hairs in one follicular unit usually exit from the same follicular ostium as closely but individually positioned 2 or 3 hair shafts. The follicular ostia correspond to the uppermost portions of the follicular epithelium known as follicular infundibula (Figure 2.1).

- Smaller empty follicular ostia and the acrosyringeal openings are visible as pinpoint white dots in skin types of IV-VI and are regularly distributed in a "starry sky" pattern (Figure 2.2).
- Bigger empty follicular ostia can also be visualized as the hypochromatic center of irregularly shaped annular structures with brown serrated borders in skin type V and VI. The center corresponds to the keratinized follicular ostium and the brown serrated outline corresponds to the more heavily pigmented infundibular epithelium (increased presence of melanin granules throughout the basal cell layer and the epidermis in darker skin) (Figure 2.3).
- Loss of follicular ostia is characteristic for scarring alopecia (Figure 2.4).
- Abnormal follicular ostia include yellow dots (dilated, usually empty ostia plugged by keratin and sebum) (Figure 2.5), peripilar sign (about 1 mm perifollicular brown halo corresponding to mild periinfundibular lymphocytic infiltrate and fine fibroplasia) (Figure 2.6), black dots (cadaverized hairs), white dots (follicular ostia replaced by fibrotic tissue), brown dots (exogenous pigmentation from anthralin) and keratotic plugs (dilated infundibula plucked by keratotic masses).

HAIR SHAFTS

The handheld dermatoscope (×10 magnification) is suitable for quick evaluation of the hair shafts and is particularly useful to detect hair weathering abnormalities and structural hair shaft abnormalities. It can estimate the approximate hair thickness (thin, intermediate or thick) but due to the small visual field more precise estimation of the ratio of the terminal:vellus hairs is difficult (the normal number of vellus hairs is up to 20%). Videodermatoscopes are equipped with software that permits measurements of the hair shaft thickness in magnified images and provides results in real scale.

- Terminal hair shafts are uniform in thickness and color (Figure 2.7). The hair fibers lie parallel to the long axis. The medulla appears as a longitudinal white band along the middle portion of the hair shaft and could be continuous, interrupted, fragmented or absent. All these are variations of normality (Figure 2.8). Fragmented medulla in individuals with thick hairs shafts is distinguished from pili annulati

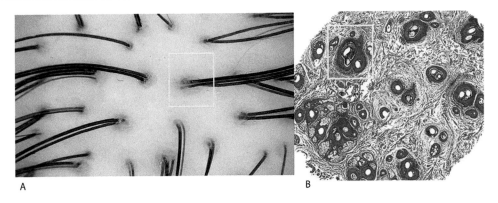

FIGURE 2.1 (A) In the normal scalp, 2 or 3 closely but individually positioned hair shafts usually exit from the same follicular ostia (×50) that are recognized on pathology (B) as follicular infundibula containing 2–3 hair shafts.

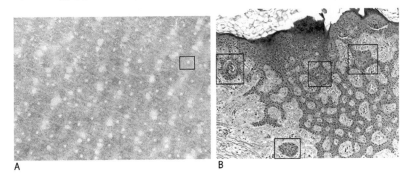

FIGURE 2.2 (A) Pinpoint white dots in a patient with alopecia universalis, skin type IV (×10); (B) they correlate to the acrosyngeal openings on pathology.

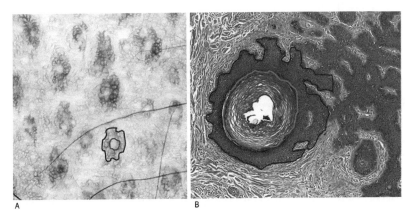

FIGURE 2.3 (A, B) Empty follicular ostia in alopecia areata in patients with skin type V-VI can show white center (keratinized follicular infundibulum) with brown serrated outline (increased presence of melanin granules throughout the basal cell layer and the epidermis in black skin).

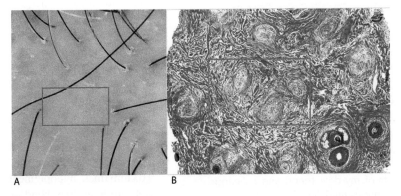

FIGURE 2.4 (A) Loss of follicular ostia in scarring alopecia (×10) corresponds to (B) follicular scarring on pathology.

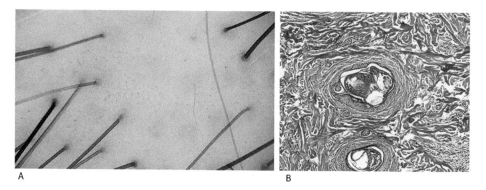

FIGURE 2.5 (A) Yellow dots (×50) correspond to (B) dilated infundibula plugged by sebum and keratin.

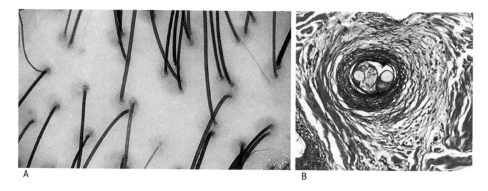

FIGURE 2.6 (A, B) Peripilar sign in androgenetic alopecia (×50) – mild periinfundubular fibroplasia with lymphocytic infiltrate.

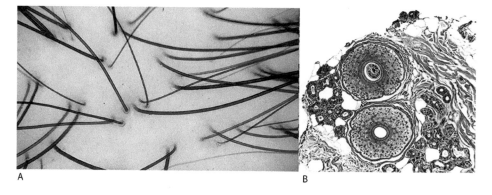

FIGURE 2.7 (A, B) Terminal hair shafts of uniform thickness (more than 0.06 mm) and color (×60). The terminal anagen follicles produce the terminal hair shafts.

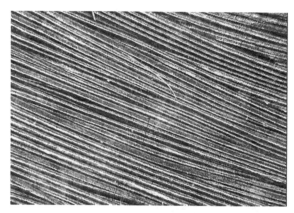

FIGURE 2.8 The hair shafts of my dear friend and colleague Dr. Giselle Martins show continuous medulla (×70).

by the fact that it affects less than 50% of the hair shaft width.

- Most hair shafts emerge as groups of 2–3 hairs known as pilosebaceous/follicular units (about 70%) (see Figure 2.6). In the frontal, temporal and occipital scalp, the majority of the follicular units show *two hairs* (45–75%), only 17–21% have three hairs and up to 40% contain single hairs, mostly located in the temporal scalp (Figure 2.9). In female pattern hair loss (FPHL), there is an increased number of follicular units with single hairs in the frontal scalp (more than 65%) (Figure 2.10).
- Thin hairs (miniaturized or vellus hairs) are less than 0.03 mm thick, hypopigmented, non-medulated, only 2–3 mm long, they bend along the axis and do not

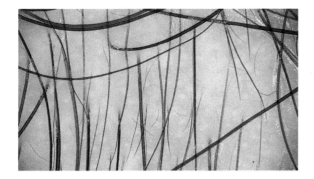

FIGURE 2.9   Single hairs in the temporal scalp (×40).

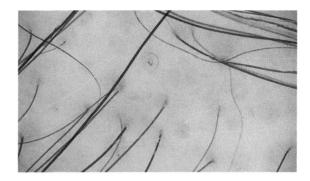

FIGURE 2.10   Single hairs and yellow dots in a woman with androgenetic alopecia, frontal scalp (×40).

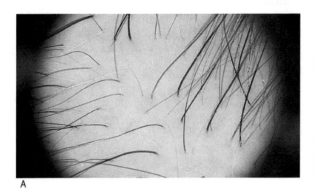

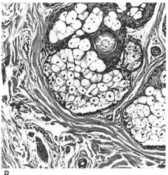

FIGURE 2.11   (A, B) Vellus hairs in androgenetic alopecia (thin hair shaft diameter). Note also the increased number of single hairs per follicular unit (×20). Vellus follicles have thin hair shafts (less than 0.03 mm) and thicker inner root sheaths.

have tapered ends compared to the upright regrowing hairs (Figure 2.11). Thin hairs account for up to 10% of all hairs. The normal number of thin hairs in the frontal and occipital area of healthy individuals is 2 per 20× field and in the temporal area is 3 per 20× field. A higher percentage (20% and above) is considered a feature of follicular miniaturization as in androgenetic alopecia and corresponds to increased number of vellus/miniaturized follicles on pathology.

• Temporal areas in women have lower hair density.

PIGMENTED NETWORK

The normal pigmented network of the scalp cannot be appreciated in fair skin individuals of Fitzpatrick skin type I-III unless they have sun exposure (Figure 2.12). In Fitzpatrick IV-VI, the normal pigmented network is presented by the honeycomb pattern, which is a uniform colored mesh of darker lines (corresponding to the pigmented basal cell layer of the rete ridges) and the hypochromatic area (corresponding to the dermal papillae) (Figure 2.13).

• White or brown patches are abnormal pigmented network in scarring alopecia in patients of Fitzpatrick skin type IV-VI and correspond to areas of fibrotic

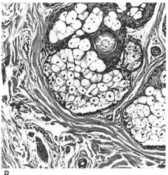

FIGURE 2.12   The normal pigmented network is irregularly enhanced in this woman with androgenetic alopecia and history of direct sun exposure (×20).

tissue replacing the follicular ostia and to postinflammatory hyperpigmentation respectively (Figure 2.14).

VASCULATURE

Rudnicka et al. have identified 18 types of blood vessel arrangements on the scalp and consider the abundance of vessels of specific morphology more indicative to the diagnosis rather than the detection of specific type of vessels.

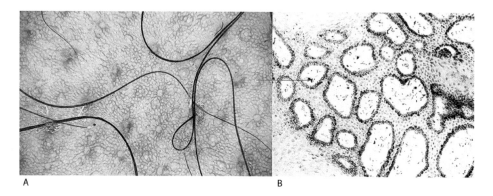

FIGURE 2.13 (A, B) Normal pigmented network in a patient of skin type V (×50): the dark lines correspond to the pigmented rete ridges and the white center corresponds to the dermal papillae (arrow) (Fontana Mason stain for melanin).

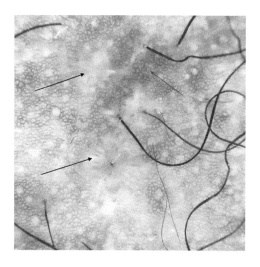

FIGURE 2.14 Abnormal pigmented network with white black arrows and dark patches red arrow in a patient with CCCA (×10).

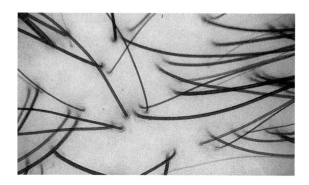

FIGURE 2.15 Dotted vessels in the normal scalp (×50).

- The normal vascular pattern of the scalp consists of dotted vessels, simple/linear red loops in the frontal and temporal scalp and thin arborizing vessels which can be found in the temporal and occipital scalp (Figures 2.15 and 2.16).
- Vessel net is a network of thin arborizing vessels forming a fine interfollicular mesh, which can be normally found in the occipital scalp and corresponds to the superficial vascular plexus with the capillary loops in the dermal papillae (Figure 2.17).

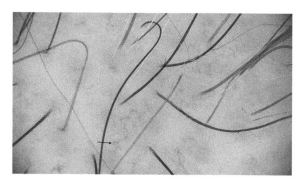

FIGURE 2.16 Thin arborizing vessels (black) and simple loops (blue) are normal findings in the frontal and temporal scalp (×50).

- Most common abnormal vascular patterns include thick arborizing vessels (discoid lupus erythematosus), glomerular vessels/twisted red loops (psoriasis), concentric perifollicular linear vessels (scarring alopecia) and enlarged irregularly bended capillaries (dermatomyositis) (Figures 2.18 and 2.19).

PEARLS

1. White hair of normal diameter is coarser and drier; therefore, applying a liberal amount of immersion liquid can help to visualize better the shafts (Figure 2.20).
2. Focal atrichia in androgenetic alopecia presents as pencil-erased areas of hair loss and can be difficult to distinguish from focal scarring alopecia. A biopsy is necessary for the diagnosis.
3. Vessels are better assessed by using videdermatoscopy at higher magnifications (×40 and up) with an immersion fluid to remove the attached scale that causes light reflection.
4. Normal scalp of prepubertal children shows dirty dots – clumped and disarrayed particulate debris 0.1–0.5 mm. They can be seen also in elderly patients in less amount. The dirty dots of the scalp

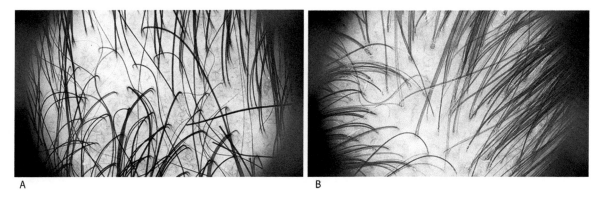

FIGURE 2.17 (A, B) Vessel net: thin vessels forming a mesh among the hairs is a normal finding on the occipital scalp of men (×20).

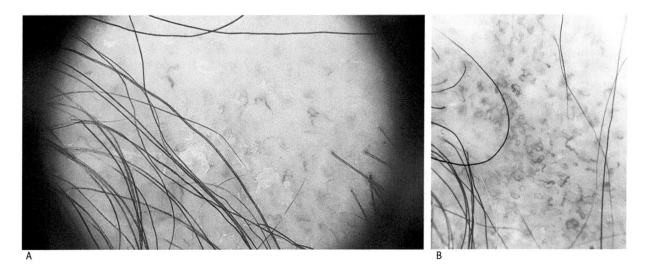

FIGURE 2.18 Abnormal tortuous/serpentine capillaries in discoid lupus erythematous (A, ×20) and (B, ×10).

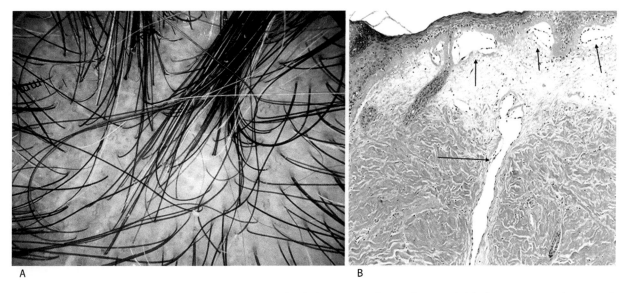

FIGURE 2.19 (A) Enlarged capillaries in dermatomyositis (×10). (Courtesy of Dr. Julio Jasso.) (B) They correspond to significantly dilated and elongated capillaries on pathology.

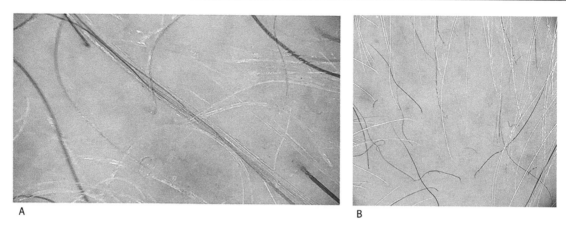

FIGURE 2.20   White hairs with minimal immersion gel (A, ×50) and with liberal immersion gel (B, ×20).

in these age groups reflect the underdevelopment/atrophy of the sebaceous gland and the absence of sebum to wash away the debris. (See Chapter 1.)

5. Improperly washed hair dye can deposit in the follicular ostia simulating black dots. The presence of the interfollicular blotches of dye can be a helpful clue.

FURTHER READING

Miteva M, Tosti A. Dermatoscopy of hair shaft disorders. J Am Acad Dermatol. 2013 Mar;68(3):473–81. doi: 10.1016/j.jaad.2012.06.041. Epub 2012 Aug 30. Review.

Rakowska A. Trichoscopy (hair and scalp videodermoscopy) in the healthy female. Method standardization and norms for measurable parameters. J Dermatol Case Rep. 2009;3(1):14–19.

Rakowska A. Trichoscopy (hair and scalp videodermoscopy) in the healthy female. Method standardization and norms for measurable parameters. J Dermatol Case Rep. 2009;3:14–9.

Rudnicka, L, Oszewska M, Rakowska A, eds. *Atlas of Trichoscopy – Dermoscopy in Hair and Scalp Disease*. 1st ed. London: Springer-Verlag; 2012:11–46.

Vincenzi C, Tosti A. Trichoscopy patterns. In: Tosti A, ed. *Dermoscopy of the Hair and Nails*. 2nd ed. Boca Raton: CRC Press; 2016:1–20.

Zhang X, Caulloo S, Zhao Y, Zhang B, Cai Z, Yang J. Female pattern hair loss: clinico-laboratory findings and trichoscopy depending on disease severity. Int J Trichology. 2012;4(1):23–28.

Practical Tips for Mastering the Scalp Biopsy Procedure

3

Giselle Martins, MD

Contents

GENERAL CONCEPTS

- The correct histologic diagnosis of alopecia requires an optimal scalp biopsy.
- It is currently known that the optimal site for the scalp biopsy should be selected by dermoscopy, particularly in scarring alopecia.
- The optimal number and size of the specimens and the location site vary among cases and will be discussed below.

SAMPLE SIZE

Scalp biopsies differ from the skin biopsies in other body areas, which can be obtained by 2–6 mm punches. The standard size for a scalp biopsy is a 4 mm punch that includes the subcutaneous tissue. The specimen can be bisected and processed as either cross sectional (horizontal) or vertical sections. Dermatologists should suggest the optimal type of bisection in their clinical request form lead by their clinical suspicion. If not specified in the request form, the dermatopathologists will process the specimen as vertical or horizontal sections depending on their level of comfort.

- Generally, two specimens are recommended for *scarring alopecia*: one for horizontal and one for vertical sections. The horizontal sections provide an overview of the follicular architecture and can identify focal disease, whereas the vertical sections visualize the dermoepidermal junction and the epidermis. If the patient agrees to have one biopsy taken only, horizontal sections should be favored.
- In *non-scarring alopecia*, usually one or two specimens are obtained and only horizontal sections are used. They have the advantage of yielding information on total number of follicles, total number of follicular units, ratio of anagen and telogen follicles, and ratio of terminal and miniaturized follicles.

DIFFUSE OR LOCALIZED ALOPECIA

The site of the scalp biopsy and the number of specimens depend on whether the dermatologist suspects diffuse or localized alopecia.

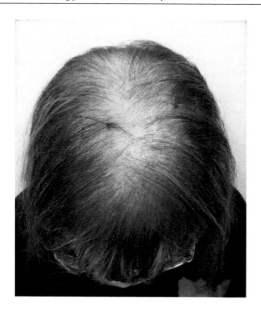

FIGURE 3.1 Avoid taking a biopsy from the mid-line part to minimize the risk of a visible small cicatrix.

In Diffuse Alopecia

- In uniform diffuse alopecia (alopecia areata incognito, chronic telogen effluvium), a single specimen from the parietal region is usually sufficient. In androgenetic alopecia, because of the parietal predilection, a single biopsy from the parietal scalp is recommended too. The mid-line part should be spared due to visibility of the scar in patients who part the hair in the middle (Figure 3.1).
- In diffuse but non-uniform alopecia (diffuse and patchy alopecia), it is suggested to obtain two biopsies, one from the parietal scalp and one from the patchy area.

In Localized Alopecia

- In localized alopecia that appears scarring, one to two specimens should be obtained from the edge of the lesion, since the center usually presents only a scar area and yields little diagnostic information to the pathologist (Figure 3.2). However, if there is a doubt that the central area may not be cicatricial (for example: cases of steroid lipoatrophy in alopecia areata may be difficult to distinguish from scarring alopecia on clinical exam and trichoscopy), a biopsy from the center is recommended too. The biopsy should be obtained using trichoscopy guidance.

In Combined Cases

Rarely two or more specimens are necessary when two or more concomitant types of alopecia are suspected (cases of frontal fibrosing alopecia associated with lichen planopilaris, and/or with diffuse alopecia areata require biopsies from frontal scalp, crown and parietal scalp, respectively).

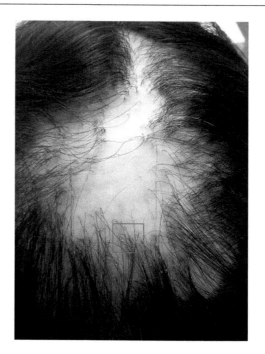

FIGURE 3.2 Localized scarring alopecia. One or two specimens including hair shafts should be obtained from the edge. In the central area, the biopsy would only show follicular scarring.

HOW TO PERFORM A SCALP BIOPSY

1. Set up the tray with all necessary instruments (Figure 3.3). It helps if the suture is already inserted in the needle holder prior to cutting out the punch as this will save time and help to achieve hemostasis faster.

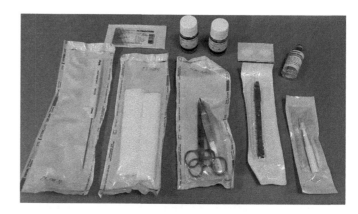

FIGURE 3.3 The biopsy tray should include: a sterile comb, some gauzes, mononylon 3.0 or 2.0 suture thread, scissors, a needle holder, Iris tweezers with teeth, a skin marking pen, a 4 mm punch and injectable anesthetic with epinephrine. The biopsy bottle is filled with formaldehyde.

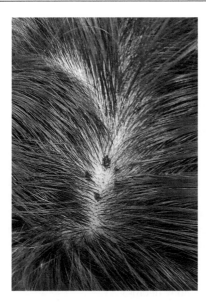

FIGURE 3.4 The selected site of the scalp biopsy is prepared by marking the area and cutting the hairs in order to facilitate the procedure.

2. Pre-choose the areas to be biopsied by using dermoscopy.
3. Mark the site with non-erasable surgical marker, so that the chosen location is visible after aseptic preparation (Figure 3.4).
4. Discuss in advance with the patient and their cardiologist if withdrawal of anticoagulant medications is possible. Ginkgo Biloba and other herbal supplements may also interfere with prolonged bleeding and should be discontinued if possible.
5. Clean the site with 70% alcohol with or without chlorhexidine. The hair from the area to be biopsied should be cut with scissors in order to facilitate the

biopsy. Long hairs wrap around the punch making it difficult to remove.
6. After choosing the site, lay the patient in a 45-degree inclination on a comfortable stretcher and anesthetize with a local anesthetic with vasoconstrictor (2% lidocaine with 1: 50.000 epinephrine), applying a volume of 0.5–1 ml per anesthetized point. The scalp is a richly vascularized region and therefore the vasoconstrictor needs time to work (about 30 minutes).

 – Younger patients bleed more than older patients whose waiting time may be shortened.
 – If the biopsied area shows dilated vessels and erythema on dermoscopy, it may be associated with more bleeding.

7. Use a 4 mm punch and rotate it only in the same direction until it reaches the subcutaneous area (Figure 3.5). For vertical sections, the punch should be inserted along the angle of the hairs to avoid transecting the follicles. For horizontal sections, this is not of importance and the punch can be inserted at a perpendicular angle. The punch should be removed gently and cut with Iris scissors without pressing the material to avoid tissue damage (Figure 3.5). Sometimes, Iris tweezers with teeth and Iris scissors are required to cut the subcutaneous tissue. The material is placed in formaldehyde to be sent to the pathology lab (Figure 3.6).
8. Mononylon 2.0 or 3.0 thread is used for the suture, which should be removed in 7 to 14 days after the procedure if it does not fall spontaneously (Figure 3.7).
9. Hydrogen peroxide and 70% alcohol with or without chlorhexidine are utilized for cleaning the site after the biopsy.

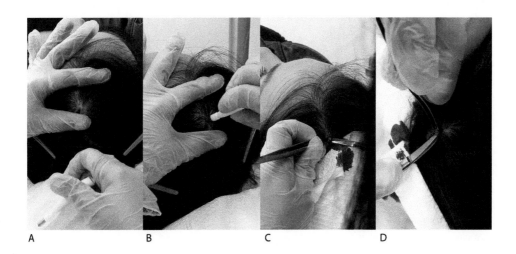

A   B   C   D

FIGURE 3.5 (A–D) Demonstration of the scalp biopsy procedure.

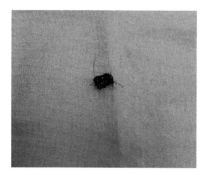

FIGURE 3.6 The obtained specimen contains the subcutaneous fat.

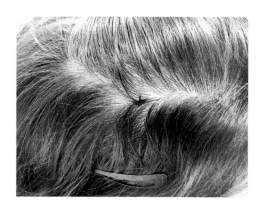

FIGURE 3.7 Mononylon 2.0 or 3.0 thread is used for the suture.

PEARLS

1. Never choose a scarred area without follicles (unless you are suspecting morphea).
2. In patchy scarring alopecia, the edges usually show signs of activity. Other good sites include perifollicular erythema and peripilar casts. Always use a dermatoscope to select the optimal area.
3. Avoid taking the specimen from areas with pustules, as the pathologist will only observe collection of neutrophils.
4. Some concomitant scalp conditions such as seborrheic dermatitis and extrafacial rosacea may unmask the optimal site for the biopsy. In these cases, it is better to treat the affected area by using shampoos and antibiotics respectively, and to proceed with the biopsy after control of the scaling is achieved. For example, if concomitant infection is not treated in lymphocytic cicatricial alopecia, the histopathological report may erroneously indicate a neutrophilic alopecia.
5. Include all relevant information in the pathology request form: patient's phototype, age, duration of hair loss, pattern (diffuse or patchy), location and trichoscopy details.

FURTHER READING

Miteva M, ed. *Alopecia*. Elsevier. Chapter 2. 2017.

Miteva M. A comprehensive approach to hair pathology of horizontal sections. Am J Dermatopathol. 2013;35(5):529–540.

Miteva M, Tosti A. Dermoscopy guided scalp biopsy in cicatricial alopecia. J Eur Acad Dermatology Venereol. 2013; 27(10):1299–1303.

Sinclair R, Jolley D, Mallari R, Magee J. The reliability of horizontally sectioned scalp biopsies in the diagnosis of chronic diffuse telogen hair loss in women. J Am Acad Dermatol. 2004;51(2):189–199.

Sperling LC, ed. *An Atlas of Hair Pathology with Clinical Correlations*. Vol. 1. New York: Parthenon Publishing Group; 2003.

Sperling LC. Scarring alopecia and the dermatopathologist. J Cutan Pathol. 2001;28(7):333–342.

Stefanato CM. Histopathology of alopecia: a clinicopathological approach to diagnosis. Histopathology. 2010;56(1):24–38.

Whiting DA. Scalp biopsy as a diagnostic and prognostic tool in androgenetic alopecia. Dermatol Ther. 1998;8:24–33.

Introduction to Horizontal Sections and Normal Scalp Anatomy on Horizontal Sections

4

Contents

GENERAL CONCEPTS

Scalp biopsies are performed in order to:

1. Diagnose scarring versus non-scarring alopecia
2. Identify the type of non-scarring alopecia based on the follicular morphology and the follicular counts and ratios in horizontal sections
3. Establish disease activity in scarring alopecia by assessing the presence and density of the inflammatory infiltrate and the extent of follicular scarring. This is particularly important for patients with scarring alopecia interested in hair transplantation

Both horizontal and vertical sections can be used to diagnose hair disorders on pathology; however, *only horizontal sections* allow for the assessment of the follicular architecture at different levels and the performance of follicular counts and ratios (Figure 4.1). Horizontal sections also allow for detecting focal scarring alopecia in patients with subtle clinical features. The concomitant use of horizontal and vertical sections in same patient enhances the diagnostic yield. However, if a single biopsy is obtained in non-scarring alopecia, it should be bisected as horizontal sections.

MOST COMMON TECHNIQUES

The Headington Technique

The most widely utilized technique was invented by John Headington in 1984 and is based on bisecting the specimen in the horizontal plane at 1 mm above the junction of the dermis/subdermis or 1 mm below the dermo-epidermal junction (Figure 4.2). This is about the level of the isthmus. The two halves are then inked at the cut side and embedded in the same block.

Step sections in the upper-half approach the epidermal surface (that allows to encompass all vellus follicles

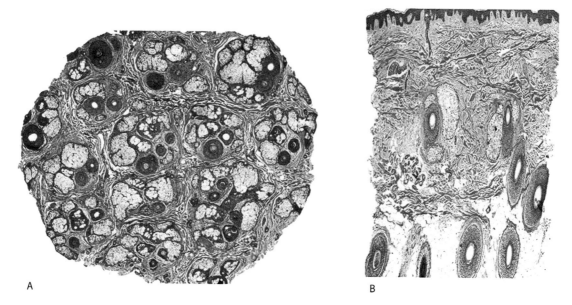

A

B

FIGURE 4.1   Horizontal sections allow for assessment of the follicular architecture and the follicular counts (A): there are 14 follicular units, 20 follicles, the terminal:vellus ratio is 1:1 and the telogen count is 40%. Vertical sections (B) show only 6 follicles and more precise follicular assessment is not possible.

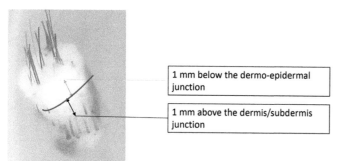

1 mm below the dermo-epidermal junction

1 mm above the dermis/subdermis junction

FIGURE 4.2   *Ex vivo* dermoscopy on a punch biopsy acquired with a handheld dermatoscope demonstrates the correct level of bisection according to the Headington technique (Handyscope, ×10).

in the follicular counts) and step sections in the lower half approach the subcutaneous fat (that allows to assess the bulbs) (Figure 4.3). If the specimen is correctly bisected, 12–20 sections are sufficient to assess the follicles at all levels and to establish a diagnosis.

Improper Bisection (Figure 4.4)

- Bisecting the specimen at the infundibular level or in the subdermis requires numerous step sections in order to reach the isthmus level (sometimes over 50). This is time and cost consuming.
- The cut is not parallel to the skin surface but tangential which results in oblique sections showing

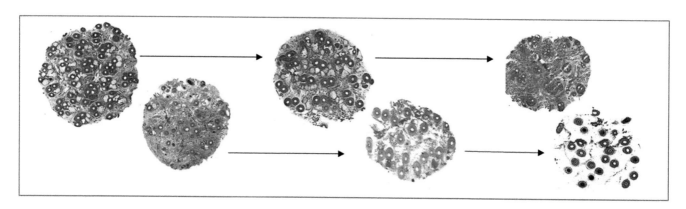

FIGURE 4.3   Horizontal sections: step sections in the upper-half approach the epidermal surface (follicular ostia) and step sections in the lower-half approach the subcutaneous fat (bulbs).

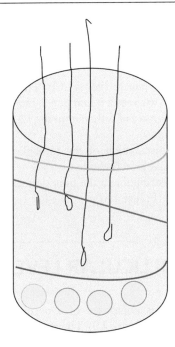

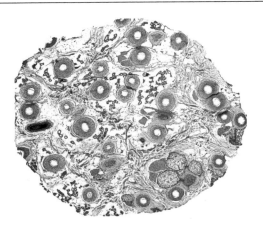

FIGURE 4.5 Tangential sections demonstrating features for lower (subcutaneous fat and sweat coils) and upper follicular levels (sebaceous glands). Care should be taken not to count the same follicles twice.

FIGURE 4.4 Schematic presentation of the incorrect bisection of horizontal sections:

- The plane of the cut is either too high, close to the surface (green) or too low, close to the subdermis (red) which can result in necessity of more than 50 sections to make the diagnosis.
- Bisection in the tangential plane (blue) and embedding the tissue tilted in the cassette can result in oblique sections with a mixture of features from several levels.

features of several levels and distorted follicular morphology (Figure 4.5). This results in inaccurate follicular counts. In some cases, the specimen needs to be even re-oriented which leads to tissue loss.

Other Techniques (Figure 4.6)

HoVert technique: the specimen is transected approximately 1 mm below the skin surface to create an epidermal disc and a lower portion. The epidermal disc is bisected and embedded in conventional fashion to obtain vertical sections. The lower portion is serially sectioned and embedded to obtain horizontal sections. This allows for simultaneous evaluation of the epidermis and the dermo-epidermal junction, and the follicular architecture with possibility to do follicular counts.

Tyler technique: the specimen is bisected first in a vertical fashion and then one half is additionally bisected in the horizontal plane. This allows for simultaneous evaluation of

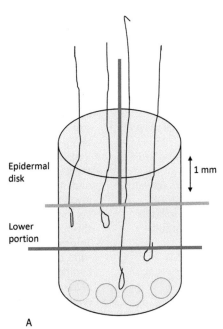

Epidermal disk

1 mm

Lower portion

A

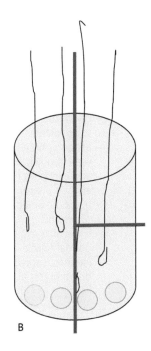

B

FIGURE 4.6 HoVert technique (A) and Tyler technique (B).

the entire specimen on vertical sections and appreciation of the follicular architecture. However, since the standard follicular counts are established in 4 mm punch specimens, this technique would not yield precise counts.

THE PILOSEBACEOUS/ FOLLICULAR UNIT

The hair follicles are intracutaneous viable epithelial structures that produce nonviable keratinized hair shafts through phases of growth, apoptosis-mediated regression (catagen) and quiescence (telogen) (see Table 4.1). The hair follicles are organized in follicular units (FU), which are best visualized at the level of the isthmus as hexagonal structures containing 3–4 terminal follicles and up to 1 vellus follicle with the attached sebaceous glands and the arrector pili muscle, surrounded by loose connective tissue (Figure 4.7). The normal number of FU in a 4 mm punch biopsy is 10–14. In scarring alopecia, the follicular units are destroyed and replaced by fibrotic tissue (follicular dropout).

PEARLS

- A 4 mm punch biopsy has circumference of 12.6 mm^2 whereas a 3 mm punch biopsy has 7 mm^2
- Normal density of follicular units: 12–14 (in a 4 mm punch biopsy)
- Orderly distribution of the follicular units at the mid-dermal level (isthmus)
- Linear distribution at the high dermal level (infundibulum) (Figure 4.8)

FOLLICULAR LEVELS

The hair follicle is composed of a permanent and a nonpermanent portion (Figure 4.9). The upper permanent portion does not cycle and includes the isthmus and infundibulum. The lower non-permanent portion is the cycling part of the follicle that reproduces the hair shaft and is made of the bulb with the dermal papilla and the suprabulbar part up

TABLE 4.1   Types of hair follicles

BASED ON THE HAIR SHAFT DIAMETER	TERMINAL	INTERMEDIATE	VELLUS
	≥0.06 mm	0.03–0.06 mm	≤0.03 mm
	– eyebrows: 5–10 mm long – eyelashes: 5–10 mm long, have the largest diameter of all body hairs	– hair after birth: rough cuticle, sparse pigmentation, fragmented medulla – early androgenetic alopecia has increased number of intermediate follicles	– non-medulated hairs, fine, non-pigmented – no attached sebaceous glands – bulbs are in the dermis – miniaturized follicles in androgenetic alopecia are often referred to as vellus follicles
BASED ON THE PHASE OF THE HAIR CYCLE	ANAGEN	CATAGEN	TELOGEN
	Follicles in growing phase (I–VI)	Follicles in transitional phase to regression	Follicles in regression
	– constitute 85–90% of all scalp follicles – anagen phase lasts 2–7 years (body hair, eyebrows and eyelashes have shorter anagen phase) – bulbs are embedded in the subdermis – show all layers of the normal follicle – inner root sheath disintegrates at the isthmus level	– less than 1% of all scalp follicles – catagen phase lasts 2–3 weeks – hair shaft retreats upwards, the outer root sheath shrinks and the follicular epithelium undergoes apoptosis	– constitute up to 15% of all scalp follicles – telogen phase lasts up to 3 months – the keratinized hair shaft undergoes degenerative involution as a serrated bright keratin mass surrounded by shrunken outer root sheath – **Telogen germina units (TGU)s** form below the club hair (fully keratinized, dead hair): basaloid palisaded epithelial strands remnants after the club hair is shed; no apoptosis at this point: this is a telogen in its end stage

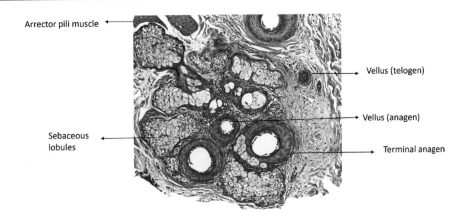

Arrector pili muscle

Vellus (telogen)

Vellus (anagen)

Sebaceous lobules

Terminal anagen

FIGURE 4.7 Follicular unit.

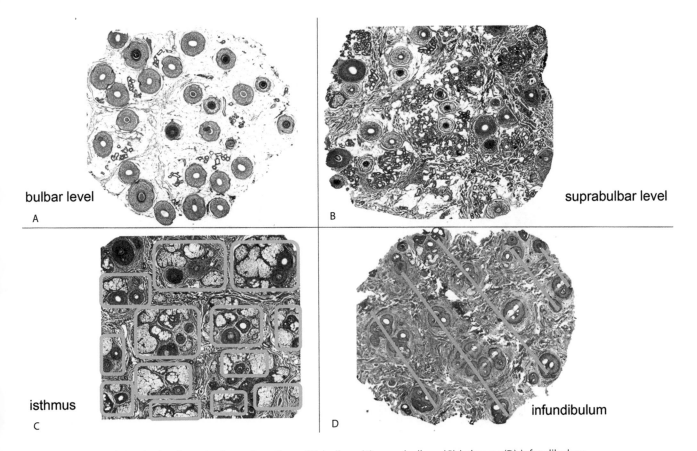

bulbar level

A

suprabulbar level

B

isthmus

C

infundibulum

D

FIGURE 4.8 The follicular levels on horizontal sections: (A) bulbar; (B) suprabulbar; (C) isthmus; (D) infundibulum.

to the Adamson fringe (that marks the upper margin of the keratogenous zone – the nucleated cells of the bulb become the anucleated cells of the stem).

- **Bulbar level** contains the bulbs randomly distributed in the fat. The bulb is composed of the matrix keratinocytes, which are rapidly proliferating cells and the hair follicle pigmentary unit (melanocytes) which surround the dermal papilla (fibroblasts and blood vessels). The papilla is formed of connective tissue in the shape of an inverted pinecone and is continuous

with the connective tissue sheath of the follicle, which terminates at the level of the infundibulum. During catagen, the dermal papilla comes into close proximity with the follicular *bulge*. On horizontal sections, the random pattern is similar to a lawn of daisies (Figure 4.10). Follicular/fibrous streamers are residual fibrovascular structures that form from the non-permanent portion at the onset of catagen and can be numerous in alopecia (normal scalp biopsies have up to 2 fibrous streamers) (Figure 4.11). They are located in the fat (for terminal follicles) and in

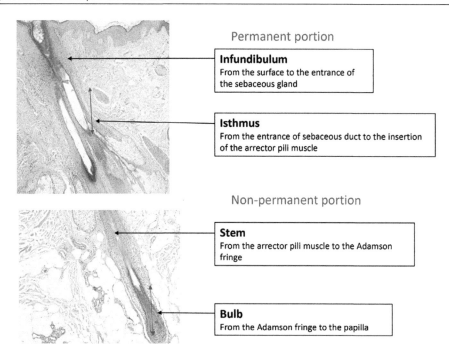

Permanent portion

Infundibulum
From the surface to the entrance of
the sebaceous gland

Isthmus
From the entrance of sebaceous duct to the insertion
of the arrector pili muscle

Non-permanent portion

Stem
From the arrector pili muscle to the Adamson
fringe

Bulb
From the Adamson fringe to the papilla

FIGURE 4.9   The portions of the hair follicle.

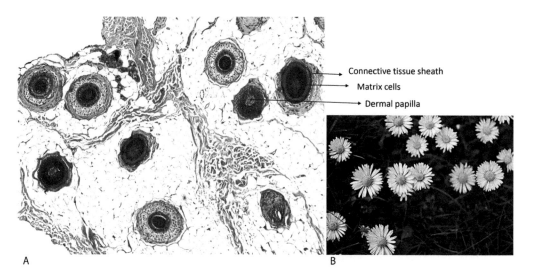

Connective tissue sheath

Matrix cells

Dermal papilla

A   B

FIGURE 4.10   (A) The bulbar level shows the random distribution of the bulbs, as in (B) a lawn of daisies.

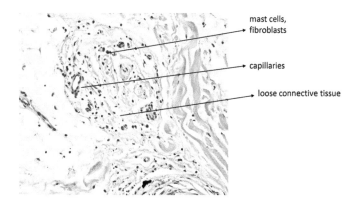

mast cells,
fibroblasts

capillaries

loose connective tissue

FIGURE 4.11 Fibrous streamers are residual fibrovascular
whorled structures.

the dermis (for vellus follicles). Fibrous streamers
may contain lymphocytes (alopecia areata), pigment
casts (alopecia areata, trichotillomania) and fragmented hairs shafts (scarring alopecia).

- **Suprabulbar level** extends approximately from the
Adamson fringe to the attachment of the arrector
pili muscle. This is the level in which the sweat coils
are located (Figure 4.12).
- **Isthmus level** contains the hair follicles organized in FU and extends from the insertion of the
sebaceous gland to attachment of the arrector pili
muscle. Each FU is surrounded by loose connective tissue that is extension of the adventitial dermis
and contains blood vessels, elastic fibers and neural

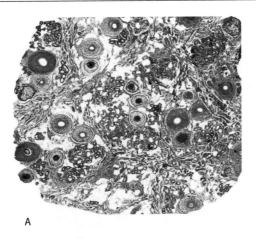
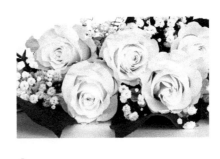

A   B

FIGURE 4.12   (A) The suprabulbar level is characterized by randomly distributed follicles, sweat coils and focal clusters of fat cells. The picture is reminiscent of (B) a bouquet of roses.

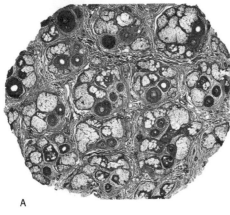
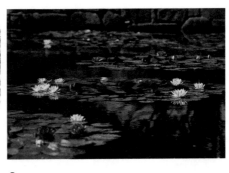

A   B

FIGURE 4.13   (A) Isthmus level: the follicular units are organized in hexagonal structures. The follicles with the attached sebaceous glands resemble (B) a pond of water lilies with their large leaves.

network. The lower isthmus contains the epithelial and melanocytic hair follicle stem cells in a small epithelial pouch called the *bulge,* which is located at the site of the insertion of the arrector pili muscle (Figures 4.13 and 4.14).

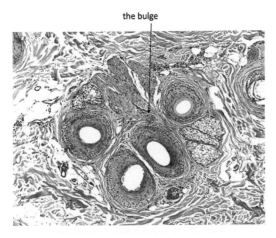

the bulge

FIGURE 4.14   This epithelial protrusion of the ORS at the level of the insertion of the arrector pili muscle is the bulge.

- **Infundibulum** is the site where 2–3 hair shafts exit the scalp through a common ostium that has the same layered structure as the interfollicular epithelium (Figure 4.15).

PEARLS

- Biopsies from individuals of African and African American ancestry show: asymmetrical follicular bulbs (twisted to one side), paired follicles and asymmetric position of the hair shaft (respectively asymmetric outer root sheath at the suprabulbar and upper follicular levels) (Figure 4.16). The paired follicles are normal findings and should not be mistaken for the compound follicles in scarring alopecia.
- The sebaceous glands undergo morphologic changes through the different ages from fully developed glands at birth (thanks to the hormonal stimulation

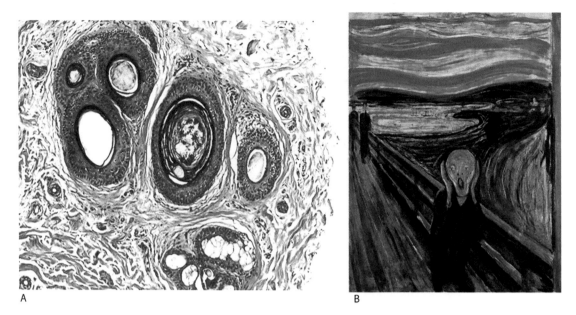

FIGURE 4.15   (A) At the infundubulm, the follicular ostia resemble skeleton or monkey faces. Note the presence of granular layer and cornified layer in the ostium in the middle. (B) The painting on the right is *The Scream* by Edvard Munch.

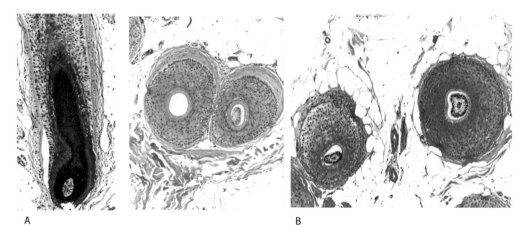

FIGURE 4.16   (A, B, C) Curved (asymmetric) bulb, paired follicles and asymmetric position of the hair shaft in scalp biopsies from African American individuals.

from the mother) through hypoplastic mantle-like epithelial structures before puberty, normal glands from puberty to adrenopause/menopause when they undergo atrophy again.

- The current concept is that the follicles from one FU share one arrector pili muscle, which contributes to maintaining follicular integrity by holding together each of the hair follicles in the FU at the isthmus level.
- The follicles of the eyebrows and eyelashes are not organized in FUs.
- The bulbs of the eyelash follicles are located in the dermis.
- Eyelash follicles lack arrector pili muscle.

ANAGEN (FIGURE 4.17)

The anagen follicle is characterized by concentric arrangements of the follicular epithelial sheaths.

- The **hair shaft/stem** (made of cuticle, cortex and medulla) is formed via migration of the cells from the hair bulb to compose the cortex. At the Adamson's fringe (the upper margin of the keratogenous zone), the nucleated hair shaft cornifies completely and gets converted to hard anucleated keratin. The Wnt signal transduction pathway is activated in normal hair follicle matrix cells to induce differentiation towards the hair shaft.

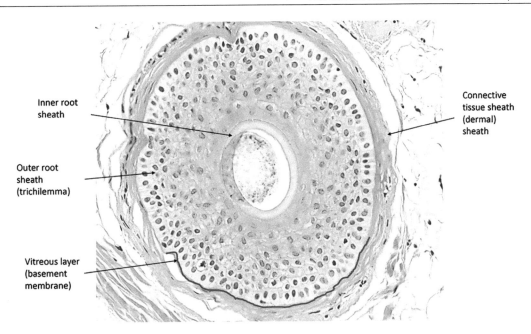

FIGURE 4.17 Anagen follicle.

- **Inner root sheath (IRS)** contains three layers: Henle's layer, Huxley layer and cuticle layer, which are not discernable on light microscopy. It anchors the hair shaft to the hair follicle tight. It undergoes abrupt (trichilemmal) keratinization and disintegrates at the isthmus level.
- **Outer root sheath (ORS)** or **trichilemma** extends from the bulb to the infundibulum where it is contiguous with the interfollicular epidermis. The ORS starts from a single layer at the tip of the bulb to become multilayered in the upper bulb. The cells of the ORS are pale due to glycogen content and begin to keratinize in a trichilemmal mode at the isthmus level. Keratinocytes in the ORS also form the *bulge* at the isthmus. The ORS contains melanocytes, Langerhans cells and Merkel cells, and key growth factors to regulate human hair follicles cycling. The ORS serves as a sleeve for the inner root sheath and the hair, which moves faster upward during anagen compared to the cells of the ORS. It is connected to the IRS (Henle's layer) via desmosomes and to the connective tissue sheath via the vitreous layer.
- **Vitreous layer (basement membrane)** is an analogical structure to the epithelial basement membrane, it separates the ORS and the connective tissue sheath.
- **Connective tissue (dermal) sheath** has two components: an outer layer of bundles of collagen arranged longitudinally and an inner one with bundles of collagen that encircle the follicle. It is composed of collagen primarily of type I, vessels and fibroblasts.

CATAGEN (FIGURE 4.18)

During catagen, the proximal part of the hair shaft keratinizes and forms the club hair, whereas the distal part of the follicle undergoes involution by apoptosis. The ORS shrinks, shows prominent individual cell apoptosis and is surrounded by a thickened vitreous layer (basement membrane).

TELOGEN (FIGURE 4.19)

The telogen club hairs are situated at the bulge level. The involuting hair shaft presents as bright and degenerated serrated keratin mass in the middle of the shrunken ORS. The telogen germinal unit (TGU) is formed below the telogen club. It is an asterisk-like structure formed by basaloid cells in a palisaded arrangement with little or no central keratinization.

Due to their morphological similarity to plants, the anagen, catagen and telogen follicles are easy to recognize in horizontal sections (Figure 4.20).

VELLUS

The vellus follicle is a "mini-version" of the terminal follicle whose bulb is situated in the mid and upper dermis. The bulb is not heavily pigmented (compared to the bulb of the terminal anagen follicle). The epithelial matrix and the dermal papilla are small. Vellus follicles/miniaturized vellus follicles cycle

apoptotic cells

Shrunken ORS

Thickened vitreous layer

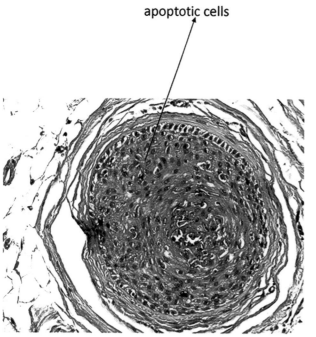

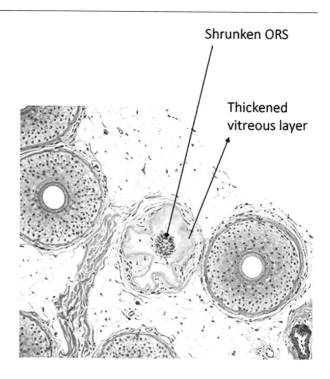

FIGURE 4.18 (A, B) Catagen follicle.

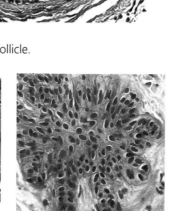

A

B

FIGURE 4.19 (A, B) Telogen follicle.

faster and therefore many of them are encountered in telogen stage in scalp biopsies (Figure 4.21).

PEARLS

- Hair follicles are in same cycle during fetal period. A few weeks after birth, the follicles enter into catagen/telogen starting from the frontal scalp. Occipital scalp follicles enter telogen in 8–12 weeks, which

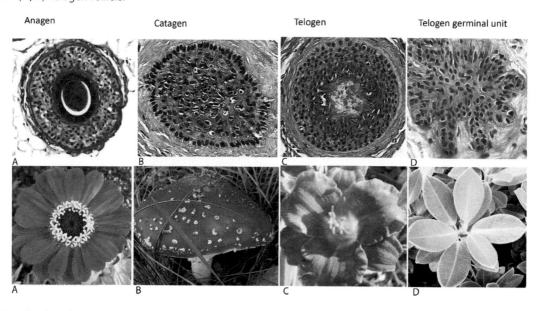

FIGURE 4.20 Visual similarity between the hair follicle types and common plants: (A) anagen; (B) catagen; (C) telogen; (D) telogen germinal unit.

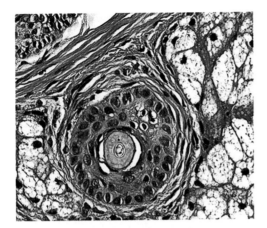

Vellus anagen: the inner root sheath is thicker than the shaft

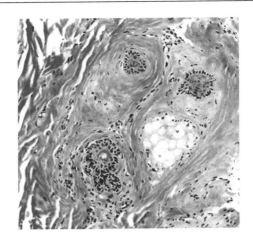

3 Vellus telogen in the upper dermis

FIGURE 4.21   (A) Vellus anagen: the inner root sheath is thicker than the shaft. (B) Vellus telogen in the upper dermis.

may result in transitory alopecia of the occipital area called neonatal transitional alopecia. Fully developed terminal follicles on scalp are present by age of 12–16 months.

- The anagen phase of eyebrow follicles is 2–3 weeks and of eyelash follicles: 4–10 weeks.
- Distinguishing terminal telogen follicles, bisected just above the level of the vestigial hair bulb and below the level of the cornified club hair from vellus telogen follicles, is difficult in horizontal sections. Vellus telogen follicles are usually situated above the level of the sebaceous glands whereas the telogen club hair is at the level of the bulge (which is lower) (Figure 4.22).
- Discrimination between anagen, catagen or telogen hairs is only possible below the bulge level.

- Catagen follicles inevitably become telogen so they are counted together with all terminal telogen follicles and TGUs.

HOW TO ASSESS HORIZONTAL SECTIONS

Assessing horizontal sections requires knowledge of the normal follicular architecture at different follicular levels and recognition of the different type of hair follicles based on their hair cycle phase and the diameter of the hair shaft.

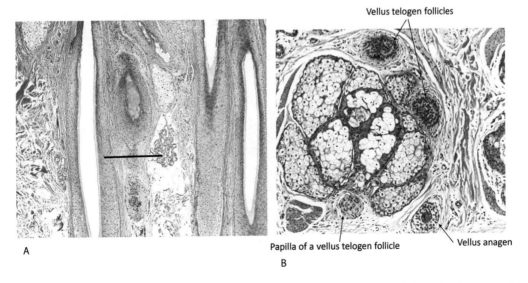

FIGURE 4.22   (A) A terminal telogen follicle, bisected just above the level of the vestigial hair bulb (level of lower isthmus). (B) The vellus telogen follicles are situated higher (level of the upper isthmus above the bulge).

Steps to build the pathological report include:

1. Assess the follicular architecture – preserved (with orderly organized follicular units at the isthmus) or altered (with areas of follicular dropout and some other features such as atrophy of the sebaceous glands).
2. Count the follicular units.
3. Count the follicles – terminal anagen, terminal telogen (count catagen, telogen and telogen germinal units together), vellus anagen and vellus telogen follicles. Fibrous streamers are counted but not added to any of the follicular counts. My opinion is that intermediate follicles should be counted together with the vellus follicles, as they inevitably become miniaturized follicles over time. One should start counting the terminal anagen follicles at the bulbar level and add additional counts (usually, 2–3 more) at the suprabulbar level and the isthmus. Terminal anagen follicles should not be counted at the infundibulum but vellus anagen follicles should be counted at the isthmus level and the infundibulum as they are rooted in the reticular and papillary

TABLE 4.2 Average normal follicular ratios and counts (4 mm punch biopsy)

Follicular units	10–14
Follicular density	38–40 (2–3.1 follicles/mm²)
Terminal anagen	31
Terminal telogen	2
Vellus	5
Fibrous streamers	2
Terminal:vellus ratio	≥4:1
Telogen count	≤15%

dermis. After counting all follicles, provide a final number for the follicular density (Figure 4.23).

4. Establish terminal:vellus ratio – (number of terminal anagen+terminal telogen) divided by (number of vellus anagen+vellus telogen follicles). (see Tables 4.2 and 4.3).
5. Establish telogen percent – (telogen count ×100) divided by (number of terminal anagen+telogen).
6. Comment on other findings such as perifollicular fibrosis, inflammatory infiltrate, fragmented hair shafts, etc.

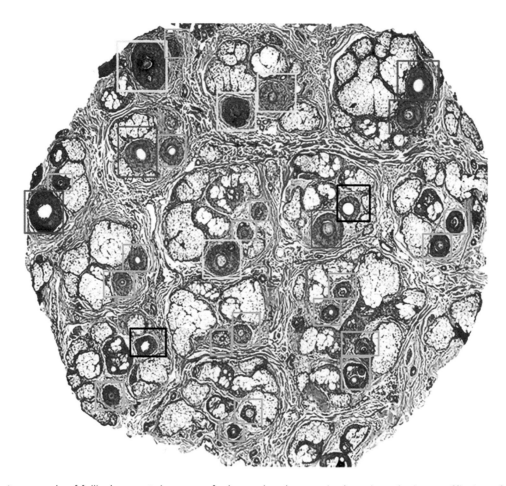

FIGURE 4.23 An example of follicular counts in a case of advanced androgenetic alopecia and telogen effluvium: follicular units 14, follicular density 27, terminal anagen (red) 5, terminal telogen (yellow) 4, vellus anagen (teal) 16, vellus telogen (teal) 2; (ratios) telogen count = 44%, terminal:vellus ratio = 0.5:1. Indeterminate follicles (black)—do not include in the count.

TABLE 4.3   Average follicular counts and ratios in most common forms of non-scarring alopecia

HAIR COUNTS	NORMAL SCALP	CHRONIC TELOGEN EFFLUVIUM	ANDROGENETIC ALOPECIA	ALOPECIA AREATA INCOGNITO
Follicular units	13	13	13	10
Terminal follicles	35	35	23	17
Vellus/Miniaturized follicles	5	4	12	8
Fibrous streamers	1–2	3	8	6
Anagen:Telogen ratio (%)	93.5:6.5	89:11	83.2:16.8	67:33
Terminal:Vellus ratio	7:1	9:1	1.9:1	3:1

PEARLS

- Follicular ratios are usually not performed in scarring alopecia.
- If only portion of the follicle is visible at the margin of a section, do not include in the counts performed for that level.
- Most data for follicular counts come from studies done in white Caucasians. Data from normal scalp biopsies of African American, Asian and Mexican populations have shown less follicular density, respectively, 22, 15 (or 1.2 follicles/mm²) and 23 follicles per 4 mm scalp biopsies. Knowing this can avoid overdiagnosing hypotrichosis/alopecia in these populations.

FURTHER READING

Elston D. The 'Tyler technique' for alopecia biopsies. J Cutan Pathol. 2012 Feb;39(2):306.

Headington JT. Transverse microscopic anatomy of the human scalp. A basis for a morphometric approach to disorders of the hair follicle. Arch Dermatol. 1984 Apr;120(4):449–56.

Lee HJ, Ha SJ, Lee JH, Kim JW, Kim HO, Whiting DA. Hair counts from scalp biopsy specimens in Asians. J Am Acad Dermatol. 2002 Feb;46(2):218–21.

Schneider MR, Schmidt-Ullrich R, Paus R. The hair follicle as a dynamic miniorgan. Cur Biol. 2009;19(3):132–142.

Miteva M Hair pathology: the basics in Alopecia, In Miteva M, ed. *Alopecia*. 1st ed. Elsevier, 2018: 23–41.

Miteva M. A comprehensive approach to hair pathology of horizontal sections. Am J Dermatopathol. 2013 Jul;35(5):529–40.

Miteva M, Lanuti E, Tosti A. Ex vivo dermatoscopy of scalp specimens and slides. J Eur Acad Dermatol Venereol. 2014 Sep;28(9):1214–8.

Nguyen JV, Hudacek K, Whitten JA, Rubin AI, Seykora JT. The HoVert technique: a novel method for the sectioning of alopecia biopsies. J Cutan Pathol. 2011 May;38(5):401–6.

Poblet E, Ortega F, Jiménez F. The arrector pili muscle and the follicular unit of the scalp: a microscopic anatomy study. Dermatol Surg. 2002 Sep;28(9):800–3.

Sperling LC. Hair density in African Americans. Arch Dermatol. 1999 Jun;135(6):656–8.

https://www.intechopen.com/books/hair-and-scalp-disorders/anatomy-and-physiology-of-hair

https://www.derm101.com/inflammatory/embryologic-histologic-and-anatomic-aspects/topography-and-regional-variation/

Trichoscopy-Guided Scalp Biopsy

5

Contents

GENERAL CONCEPTS

The idea behind using the dermatoscope to select the optimal site for the scalp biopsy is similar to that of using an imaging technique to guide obtaining the optimal tissue sample (for instance, using the ultrasound transducer to guide the needle insertion for fine needle aspiration in a solid tumor mass). Any handheld dermatoscope or videodermatoscope can be used for the purpose of the dermoscopy-guided biopsy. Most practical is the use of a handled dermatoscope attached to a camera such as Dermlite (3 Gen LLC, USA) or the Handyscope (FotoFinder Systems, Bad Birnbach, Germany) attached to the iPhone (Apple, Cupertino, CA, USA). Both devices allow capturing dermoscopic images and zooming in on details in high magnification. The selected area is outlined by a surgical pen and can be photographed again to provide the pathologist with the exact correlate for the histologic findings.

This approach has several advantages:

1. Non-invasive, fast and cost-effective
2. Helps the clinician to detect and biopsy areas of early/focal scarring alopecia
3. Allows studying the morphology of special features of interest (such as flame hairs, pinpoint white dots and others, see Chapter 1)

MAIN USES

In Scarring Alopecia

This approach is most useful for optimizing the diagnostic yield of the biopsy in cases of suspected scarring alopecia. The biopsy should be taken from a diagnostic area and not from an area with already existing scarring (Figure 5.1, Table 5.1).

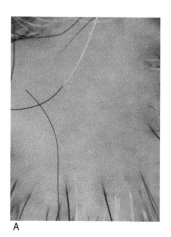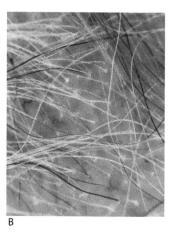

A   B

FIGURE 5.1 The biopsy should be taken from an area with activity as shown in (B) and not from a scarred area (A) (×10).

In Non-Scarring Alopecia

The value of the trichoscopy-guided approach is usually restricted to the patchy type of alopecias, which show variety of trichoscopic morphology. Diffuse non-scarring alopecia in women does not require trichoscopy as the biopsy site is standard – the parietal scalp or the crown. An exception consists of clinically apparent small (less than 0.5 × 0.5 cm) hairless patches in an otherwise classic, usually longstanding androgenetic alopecia that should be biopsied to exclude androgenetic alopecia with focal atrichia versus Fibrosing Alopecia in a Pattern Distribution (FAPD). Polarized microscopy can help distinguish the areas of focal atrichia in AGA from follicular scars in scarring alopecia as the latter contain compact collagen that would be positive under polarized light and the fibrous streamers remain negative (see also Androgenetic Alopecia). (See Table 5.2.)

TABLE 5.1 Optimal site for obtaining the scalp biopsy in scarring alopecia (Figures 5.2–5.14)

HAIR DISORDER	TRICHOSCOPY FEATURES FOR OPTIMAL SITE OF BIOPSY	HISTOLOGIC CORRELATION
Lichen planoilaris (LPP)	Individual or compound hairs with peripilar (concentric or tubular white) casts	Individual or compound follicular structures (fused follicles) surrounded by perifollicular fibrosis and lichenoid inflammation
Frontal fibrosing alopecia (FFA)	Single hairs with peripilar casts	Follicles surrounded by perifollicular fibrosis and lichenoid inflammation
	Single hairs with peripilar hypopigmentation	
	Hairs with transparent proximal hair emergences in the preauricular area Eyebrows: broken hairs	
Fibrosing alopecia in a pattern distribution (FAPD)	Individual or compound hairs with peripilar concentric or tubular casts	Individual or compound follicular structures (fused follicles) surrounded by mild perifollicular fibrosis and lichenoid inflammation, involving the vellus follicles
Discoid lupus erythematosus (DLE)	Keratotic plugs	Dilated infundibula plugged by keratin
	Follicular red dots	Perifollicular lymphoid cell infiltrate with dilated vessels and red blood cell extravasation at the level of the upper follicle
	Speckled blue-gray dots Blue-white veil	Interface vacuolar damage at basement membrane of the follicular epithelium with pigment incontinence
Dissecting cellulitis of the scalp	3D yellow dots	Dilated follicular ostia plugged by keratin and sebum
	Broken hairs	Telogen follicles surrounded by dense mixed cell inflammation
Folliculitis decalvans	Tufts of 6 or more hairs emerging from the same ostium surrounded by white-yellowish scales	Multi-compound follicular structures with perifollicular fibrosis, and lichenoid and interstitial mixed cell infiltrate
Central centrifugal cicatricial alopecia (CCCA)	One or two hairs emerging together, surrounded by white/gray halo	Compound hair follicles with lichenoid infiltrate and more prominent perifollicular fibrosis
Tinea capitis	Comma hairs Broken hairs Corkscrew hairs	Hair shafts with fungal spores
Acute traction alopecia	Broken hairs	Hair follicles showing features for trichomalacia and pigmented casts

Lichenoid infiltrate   Perifollicular fibrosis

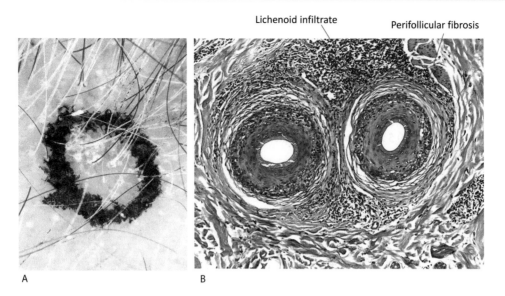

FIGURE 5.2 (A, B) Individual hairs or compound hairs with peripilar white casts are selected by trichoscopy (×20). They correspond to individual or compound follicular structures (fused follicles) surrounded by perifollicular fibrosis and lichenoid inflammation in lichen planopilaris and frontal fibrosing alopecia.

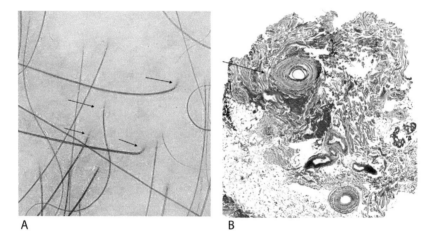

FIGURE 5.3 (A) Hairs with transparent proximal hair emergences in the preauricular area in FFA (×20) correspond to affected follicles with perifollicular fibrosis and lichenoid infiltrate (B).

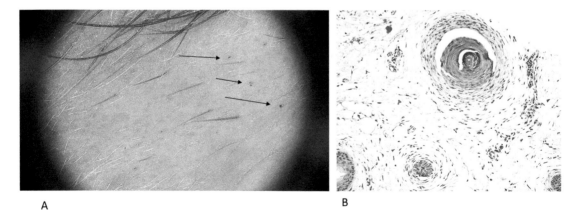

FIGURE 5.4 (A) Black dots and broken hairs among pink dots in eyebrow FFA (×20). On pathology, there is perifollicular fibrosis and mild perifollicular lichenoid inflammation (B).

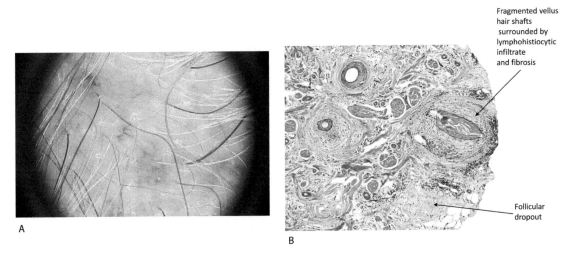

FIGURE 5.5 (A) Fibrosing alopecia in a pattern distribution: biopsy is taken from the hairs with peripilar casts. Note the hair shaft variability (×20). (B) On pathology, there are areas of follicular dropout. There is perifollicular fibrosis and lichenoid inflammation surrounding vellus follicles.

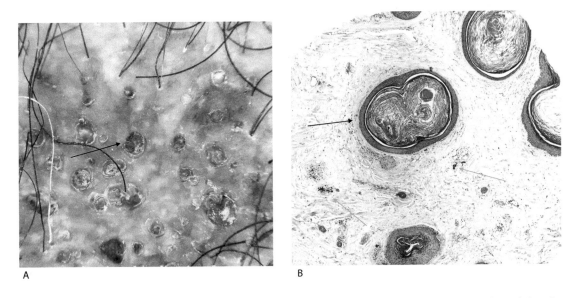

FIGURE 5.6 (A) Keratotic plugs in discoid lupus erythematosus (×20). (B) Note the pale stroma with mucin and the pigment incontinence on histology (blue arrows).

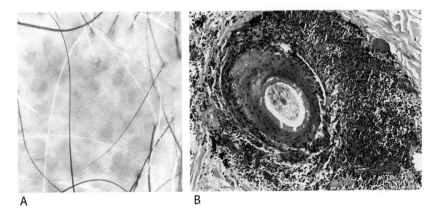

FIGURE 5.7 (A) Follicular red dots in DLE (×10) correspond to perifollicular lymphoid cell infiltrate with dilated vessels and red blood cell extravasation (B).

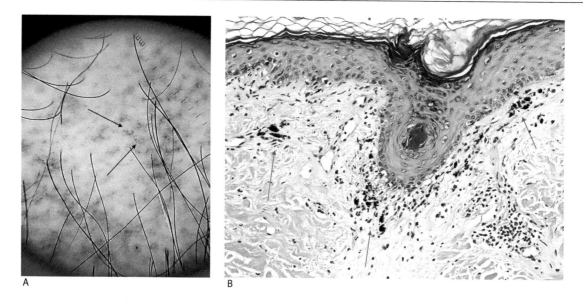

FIGURE 5.8 (A) The speckled blue-gray dots (×10) correspond to interface vacuolar damage at basement membrane of the follicular epithelium with pigment incontinence (red) (B).

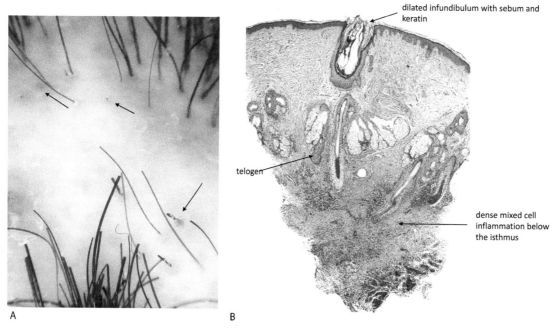

dilated infundibulum with sebum and keratin

telogen

dense mixed cell inflammation below the isthmus

FIGURE 5.9 (A) 3D yellow dots and broken hairs in dissecting cellulitis of the scalp (×10) corresponding to dilated infundibula plugged by sebum and keratin, and to telogen follicles in a "sea" of inflammation (B).

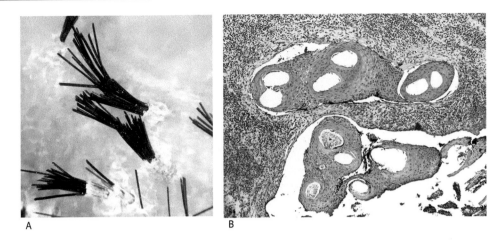

FIGURE 5.10   (A) Tufts of more than 6 hairs coming from the same ostium surrounded by white tubular casts (×10) correspond to compound follicular structures (fused follicles), surrounded by mixed cell infiltrate of neutrophils, plasma cells and lymphocytes (B).

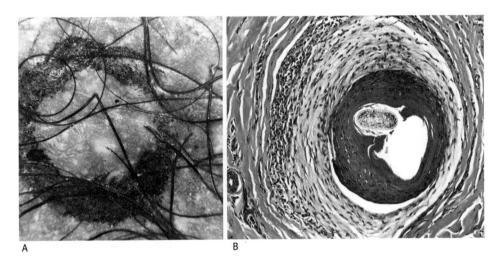

FIGURE 5.11   (A) Peripilar white-gray smooth halo in CCCA (×10) corresponds to the concentric perifollicular fibrosis with/without lichenoid inflammation surrounding compound follicles at the level of the isthmus and above (B).

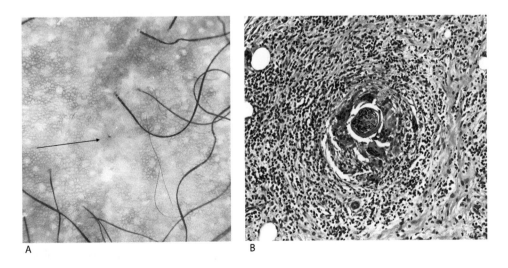

FIGURE 5.12   (A) A broken hair on a background of milky white areas in CCCA (×10) corresponds to a destroyed follicle with dense – in this case, granulomatous – inflammatory infiltrate (B).

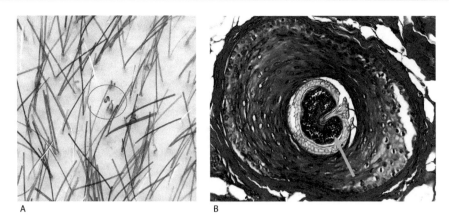

FIGURE 5.13 The comma hair (×10) (circle on A) corresponds to infected hair shafts loaded with fungal spores (arrow on B).

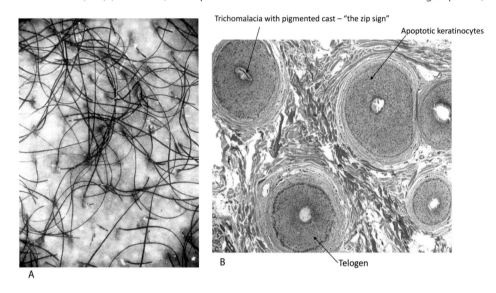

FIGURE 5.14 (A) Numerous broken hairs in acute traction alopecia in a patient who removed a glued wig (×10). They correspond to follicles undergoing catagen/telogen with trichomalacia and pigmented casts (B).

TABLE 5.2 Trichoscopic-pathologic correlation in non-scarring alopecia (Figures 5.15–5.19) (see also Chapter 2)

HAIR DISORDER	TRICHOSCOPY FEATURES FOR OPTIMAL SITE OF BIOPSY	HISTOLOGIC FEATURES
Alopecia areata	Yellow dots Cadaverized hairs Dystrophic hairs Exclamation hairs	Usually empty, dilated infundibula plugged by sebum and loose keratin Telogen follicles "Swarm of bees" infiltrate at the bulbar level
Trichotillomania	Broken hairs: *Flame hair* *Tulip hair* *Hair powder* *V-sign* *Coiled hair*	Hair shafts affected by trichomalacia and pigmented casts
Pressure induced alopecia	Black dots Broken hairs	Telogen follicles
Lichen simplex chronicus	Broom-like hairs	Affected hair shafts revealing the hamburger sign
Androgenetic alopecia (AGA) with focal atrichia	Small hairless patches	Focal follicular dropout with non-cycling "frozen" fibrous streamers

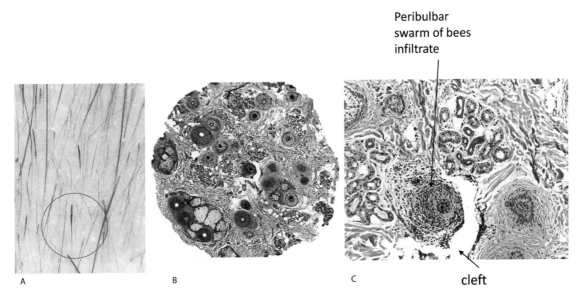

FIGURE 5.15 (A) An example of dystrophic hair in alopecia areata (exclamation hair) (×10) that was sampled with a 1 mm punch biopsy inserted within the 4 mm punch specimen (B) (note the cleft from the 1 mm punch cut in the tissue) around a telogen follicle with a swarm of bees infiltrate (C).

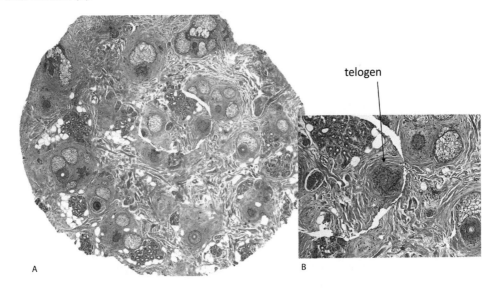

FIGURE 5.16 (A) Another example of a dystrophic hair in alopecia areata, sampled by 1 mm punch inserted in the 4 mm punch specimen, corresponds to a telogen follicle (B).

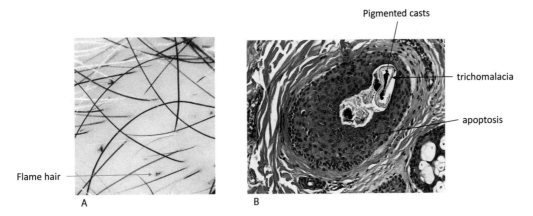

FIGURE 5.17 (A) The broken hairs in trichotillomania correspond to trichomalacia (distorted hair shaft), pigmented casts and many apoptotic cells in the outer root sheath (a catagen involution) (B).

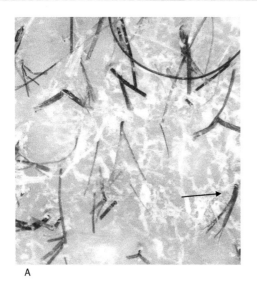
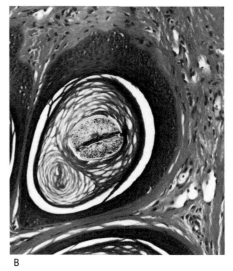

A   B

FIGURE 5.18   (A) Broom-like hairs in lichen simplex chronicus (×10) correspond to traumatically split hair shafts forming the hamburger sign (B).

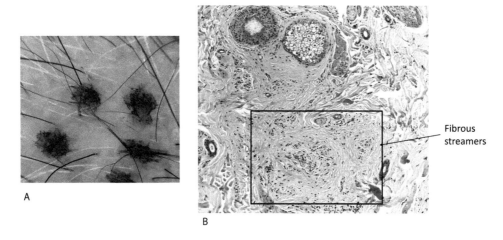

A

B

FIGURE 5.19   (A) A small area that appears hairless (focal atrichia) in this case of AGA is encircled for a trichoscopy-guided biopsy (×10). The focal atrichia corresponds to focal areas of follicular dropout consisting of non-cycling fibrous streamers (B).

FURTHER READING

Miteva M, Tosti A. Dermoscopy guided scalp biopsy in cicatricial alopecia. J Eur Acad Dermatol Venereol. 2013 Oct;27(10):1299–303.

Miteva M, Tosti A. Polarized microscopy as a helpful tool to distinguish chronic nonscarring alopecia from scarring alopecia. Arch Dermatol. 2012 Jan;148(1):91–4.

Miteva M. Hair Pathology: the basics. In Miteva M, ed. *Alopecia*. 1st ed. Elsevier; 2018:23–41.

Quaresma MV, Mariño Alvarez AM, Miteva M. Dermatoscopic-pathologic correlation of lichen simplex chronicus on the scalp: 'broom fibres, gear wheels and hamburgers'. J Eur Acad Dermatol Venereol. 2016 Feb;30(2):343–5.

Clues to Pathologic Diagnosis of Hair Disorders

6

Contents

GENERAL CONCEPTS

"A *clue* is something that guides through an intricate procedure or maze of difficulties, specifically: a piece of evidence that leads one toward the solution of a problem" (as per Merriam-Webster Dictionary).

Several obstacles in diagnosing scalp biopsies prompted the search for helpful clues:

1. The anatomical complexity of the pilosebaceous structures in various stages of the hair cycle on horizontal sections
2. Suboptimal 2 or 3 mm punch biopsies are difficult to interpret when it comes to hair loss because there is no sufficient number of follicular units for assessment of the architecture and the pattern (exception – small 2–3 mm trichoscopy-guided scalp biopsies are acceptable in frontal fibrosing alopecia).
3. Suboptimal processing of the specimen with features for several follicular levels in the same section.
4. The difficulty to perform clinico-pathological correlation based on a 2–3 mm punch biopsy bisected vertically and a clinical rule out diagnosis of diffuse non-scarring alopecia, for example.

Simple clues for the histologic diagnosis of hair disorders are therefore needed. However, histologic clues are not diagnostic criteria and it is the process of connecting the clues and correlating them to the provided clinical information, rather than relying on a single clue to make a correct diagnosis. Nonetheless, when definitive diagnosis is not feasible for many reasons, including the obstacles outlined above, it is better to describe the findings, rather than speculate on a single diagnosis that can result in prolonged and inaccurate treatments.

Some helpful clues are outlined here (see also Chapter 4).

PATIENT'S ETHNICITY

Patient's ethnicity can be a helpful clue to the diagnosis of scarring alopecia, as some disorders such as traction alopecia (TA) and central centrifugal cicatricial alopecia (CCCA) are more prevalent in or exclusive to African Americans. Clues in scalp biopsies from African Americans include:

- Follicular asymmetry including asymmetric (twisted) bulb and asymmetric position of the hair shaft at the level of the mid and upper follicle. The shape of the follicle is helical (spiral) whereas in Caucasians and Asians, it is straight (Figure 6.1). The axial

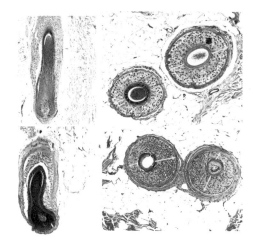

FIGURE 6.1 The top row shows a straight follicular bulb and equidistant positioning of the hair shaft (symmetric outer root sheath) in a Caucasian. Compare with the twisted bulb and asymmetrically positioned hair shaft in an African American (low row). Note also that the follicles are paired with approximate connective tissue sheaths in African Americans.

asymmetry and the helical shape lead to points of geometric weakness of the intrafollicular portion of the hair shaft. The geometric sites of weakness together with the thinner cuticle, in the setting of inflammation and/or trauma lead to easier hair breakage and migration of the hair shafts through the follicular epithelium in the stroma (Figure 6.2).

- Paired hair follicles: two adjacent follicles lie close to each other and "connect" by their connective tissue sheaths (see Figure 6.1).
- It is also common to see melanophages in the dermis and this should not be misinterpreted as an abnormal finding (Figure 6.3).

PATIENT'S AGE

- *Prepubertal children* do not have well-developed sebaceous glands. In the newborn, the sebaceous gland is fully developed and involutes in the following months due to the drop of maternal androgens to become *a mantle*: cords of epithelial cells emanating

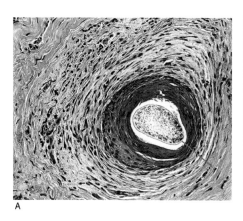

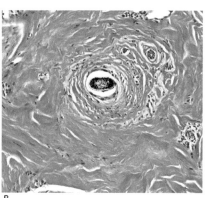

FIGURE 6.2 (A) The asymmetric position of the hair shaft and thinner cuticle enable (B) easier destruction of the follicle at sites of geometric weakness (arrow) and migration of the hair shaft into the dermis.

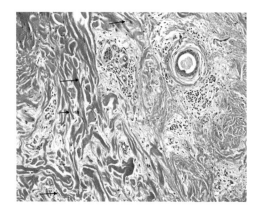

FIGURE 6.3 Melanophages in the dermis are normal finding in scalp biopsies from African Americans.

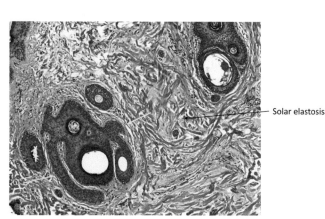

Solar elastosis

FIGURE 6.4 Sebaceous glands present as immature/atrophic mantle-like structures in prepubertal children and in elderly individuals.

from both sides of the hair follicle at its upper level. In horizontal sections, this is observed as cords "embracing" the follicles. During *menopause/andropause* when the androgens drop the sebaceous glands acquire the mantle appearance again (Figure 6.4).

CLUES IN NON-SCARRING ALOPECIA

- Fibrous streamers (FS, follicular stelae) in the lower dermis and subdermis indicate terminal catagen or telogen follicles whereas FS detected only in the mid- or upper dermis indicate vellus catagen or telogen follicles (vellus follicles are rooted and cycle in the dermis). Therefore, an increased number of FS in the upper dermis is a clue to follicular miniaturization (Figure 6.5).

- A significantly decreased number of follicular bulbs in the subdermis is a clue to androgenetic alopecia. Due to follicular miniaturization, the miniaturized follicles cycle in the dermis (see Figure 6.5).
  Caveat: Chronic stage alopecia areata and permanent alopecia after chemotherapy may show a similar pattern.
- *Zip and button signs* correspond to aberrant aggregation of the cortical melanin granules either as a vertical streak or as a centrally located clump in hair follicles with disrupted morphology due to follicular injury or trauma (a clue to trichotillomania and acute traction alopecia) (Figure 6.6).
- Pigmented casts in the follicular canal associated with vellus hair favor alopecia areata over trichotillomania – in trichotillomania, the vellus hairs are spared from trauma (Figure 6.7).
- *Hamburger sign*: vertically oriented split in the hair shaft containing proteinaceous material and red blood

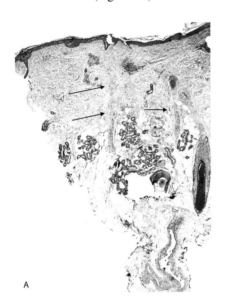
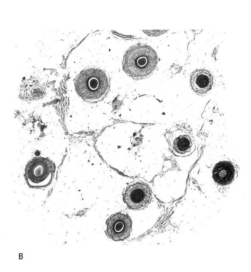

A   B

FIGURE 6.5 (A) Fibrous streamers in the dermis and only few follicular bulbs in the fat (empty fat) (B) are clues to follicular miniaturization.

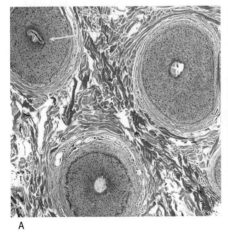
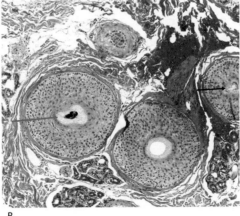

A   B

FIGURE 6.6 Zip (A, yellow arrow) and button sign (B, blue arrow) in acute traction alopecia and trichotillomania (compare with the normally distributed melanin granules in the cortex of a normal hair shaft (B, black arrow).

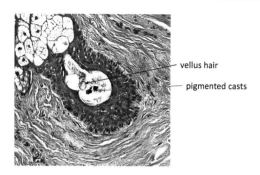

FIGURE 6.7 Pigmented casts associated with vellus follicles is a clue to alopecia areata versus trichotillomania. (From Miteva et al. Am J Dermatopathol. 2014 Jan;36(1):58–63 with permission.)

cells is a clue to trichotillomania, trichoteiromania and lichen simplex chronicus (LSC). Sometimes, the hair shafts are fragmented in more pieces – "hamburger crumbs". In LSC, this sign is associated with *gear wheel-like follicular structures* at the level of the infundibulum, which correspond to the jagged acanthosis of the follicular epithelium (Figure 6.8).

- A "swarm of bees" infiltrate refers to lymphocytes, dendritic cells and natural killer (NK) cells in the peribulbar area of the anagen hair follicle and is a clue to the diagnosis of acute stage alopecia areata (Figure 6.9). *Caveat:* The "swarm of bees" infiltrate can also be seen in syphilitic alopecia associated with widened infundibular ostia and pigmented casts.

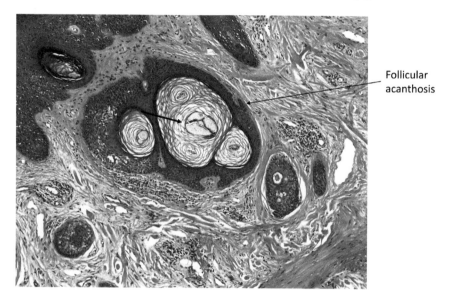

FIGURE 6.8 Hamburger sign in lichen simplex chronicus.

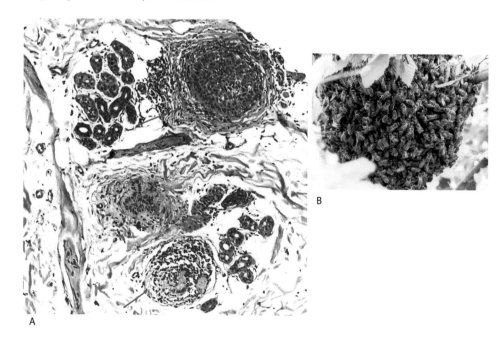

FIGURE 6.9 (A) Alopecia areata at the bulbar level displaying swarm of bees infiltrate (arrows) (B). The infiltrate affects terminal follicles.

CLUES IN SCARRING ALOPECIA

- *Eyes and goggles:* groups of two follicles in compound structures (compound follicles/follicular packs) are a clue to scarring alopecia. The *eyes* resemble the eyes of an owl with big circles of feathers around the eyes; the *goggles* resemble aviator's or swimmer's goggles. *Owl eyes* are seen when the fusion occurs between the connective tissue sheaths of the follicles. The hair shaft with its inner root sheath (if present) looks like the eye (pupil and iris), and the outer root sheath, the concentric fibrosis and the lichenoid infiltrate look like the big concentric circles of feathers around each owl's eye (Figure 6.10). In the *goggles,* the fusion is between the outer root sheaths of the fused follicles and the concentric fibrosis with the lichenoid infiltrate encircling the entire goggles (Figure 6.11). In the eyes, the follicles still maintain their individuality whereas in the goggles – they become a united follicular structure: they lose their individuality.

Caveat: The eyes and goggle sign should not be confused with normal infundibular structures, which contain two three follicles. This sign should be evaluated at the level of the isthmus and below (see Figure 6.11).

- *Number of compound follicles (follicular packs):* two packs are a clue to lymphocytic cicatricial alopecia whereas four or five follicular packs highly suggest neutrophilic cicatricial alopecia; with six or more follicular packs "monster goggles", the diagnosis of neutrophilic cicatricial alopecia is nearly certain. (Figure 6.12).
- *Hair shafts* in FS is a clue to scarring alopecia. They are a sign of follicular destruction and hair breakage in the follicular canal and they can consist of intact hair shafts (with preserved cuticle) or fragments of hair shafts. They are most commonly detected in CCCA but are not specific. In neutrophilic cicatricial alopecia, fragmented hairs shafts are usually detected "naked" within granulomas (Figure 6.13).
- *Follicular triad* is the concomitant involvement of vellus, terminal anagen and telogen follicles by

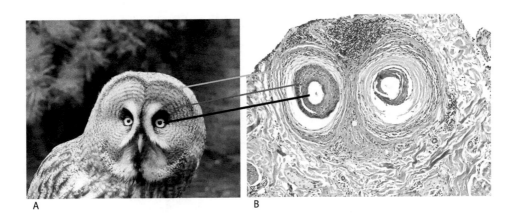

FIGURE 6.10   (A) Owl eyes in (B) frontal fibrosing alopecia.

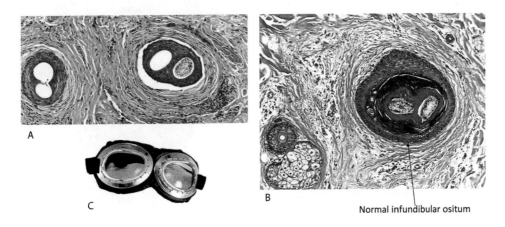

Normal infundibular ositum

FIGURE 6.11   (A) Lichen planopilaris displaying the goggles clue (C). The normal infundibular ostia contain 2 or 3 hair shafts (B) and should not be mistaken for the eyes and goggles in scarring alopecia.

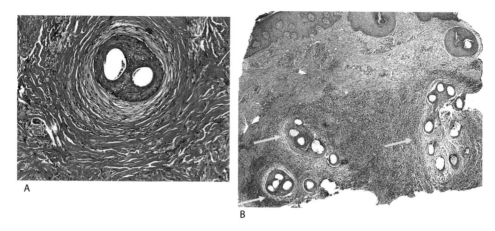

FIGURE 6.12 (A) Two packs (goggles) are a clue to lymphocytic cicatricial alopecia and (B) "monster goggles" (6-packs) are a clue to neutrophilic cicatricial alopecia (yellow arrows).

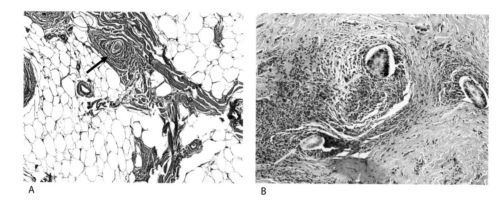

FIGURE 6.13 Fragmented (naked) hair shafts in fibrous streamers in central centrifugal cicatricial alopecia (black arrow) (A) and fragmented hair shaft with granulomatous inflammation in the dermis in folliculitis decalvans (B, yellow arrows).

lichenoid inflammation and perifollicular fibrosis and is a clue to FFA. Generally, vellus follicles are considered an early target in FFA. The persistence of the lichenoid infiltrate around catagen/telogen follicles may be due to the increased apoptotic activity in the outer root sheaths, which switches faster the affected follicles from anagen to catagen (Figure 6.14).

- Dense mixed cell infiltrate extending at all follicular levels (from the upper dermis through the subdermis) is a clue to inflammatory tinea capitis (tinea-capitis mimicking dissecting cellulitis of the scalp). Dense mixed cell infiltrate restricted to the lower dermis, below the isthmus level, favors dissecting cellulitis of the scalp. (Figure 6.15).
- Syringoma-like structures are dilated eccrine ducts and are a clue to scarring alopecia. Most likely, they form in the setting of altered follicular architecture and increased traction forces from the fibrosis in the stroma (Figure 6.16). In my experience, they are more common in CCCA, however they are not specific.

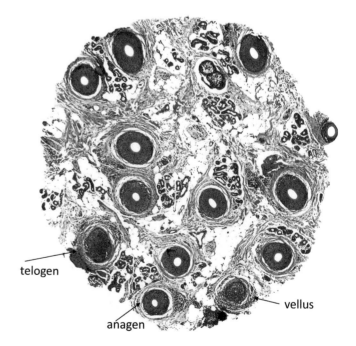

telogen

vellus

anagen

FIGURE 6.14 Follicular triad (involvement of vellus, terminal anagen and telogen follicles by lichenoid infiltrate and fibrosis) in FFA.

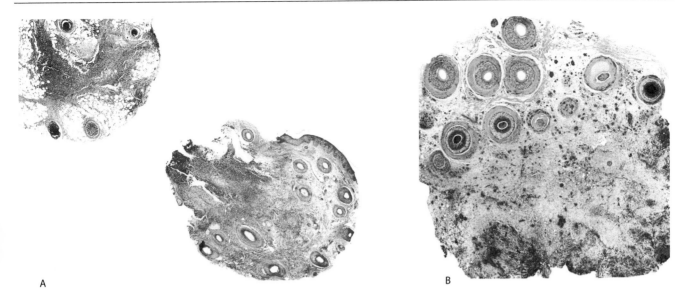

FIGURE 6.15 (A) Dense mixed cell inflammatory infiltrate involving the entire dermis and subdermis in inflammatory tinea capitis versus (B) predilection of similar infiltrate for the lower dermis and subdermis in dissecting cellulitis of the scalp.

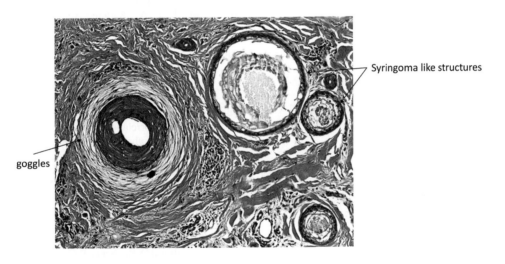

FIGURE 6.16 Dilated ducts (syringoma-like structures) in CCCA.

MISCELLANEOUS CLUES

- Lymphocytes in perineural distribution is a clue to morphea/linear morphea *en coup de sabre* of the scalp (Figure 6.17).
- Plasma cells in FS is a clue to psoriatic alopecia secondary to tumor necrosis factor-alpha inhibitors and to syphilitic alopecia (Figure 6.18).
- Collections of plasma cells in the subdermis are a clue to the diagnosis of syphilitic alopecia, tinea capitis, neutrophilic cicatricial alopecia such as folliculitis decalvans and to lupus panniculitis.

FURTHER READING

Doyle LA, Sperling LC, Baksh S, Lackey J, Thomas B, Vleugels RA, Qureshi AA, Velazquez EF. Psoriatic alopecia/alopecia areata-like reactions secondary to anti-tumor necrosis factor-α therapy: a novel cause of noncicatricial alopecia. Am J Dermatopathol. 2011 Apr;33(2):161–6.

Kazakov, D., et al., eds. *Cutaneous Adnexal Tumors.* Wolters Kluwer/ Lippincort Williams & Wilkins: Philadelphia; 2012:333–37.

Lindelöf B, Forslind B, Hedblad MA, Kaveus U. Human hair form. Morphology revealed by light and scanning electron microscopy and computer aided three-dimensional reconstruction. Arch Dermatol. 1988 Sep;124(9):1359–63.

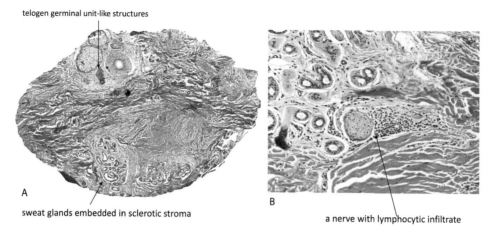

telogen germinal unit-like structures

A

sweat glands embedded in sclerotic stroma

B

a nerve with lymphocytic infiltrate

FIGURE 6.17   Scalp morphea (A, B). Lymphocytes in a perineural distribution (B) can be a helpful clue to the diagnosis.

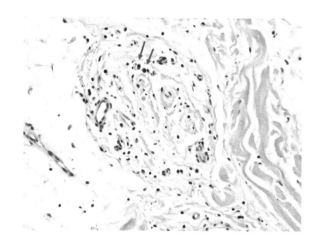

FIGURE 6.18   Plasma cells in fibrous streamers in a case of syphilitic alopecia.

Miteva M, Torres F, Tosti A. The 'eyes' or 'goggles' as a clue to the histopathological diagnosis of primary lymphocytic cicatricial alopecia. Br J Dermatol. 2012 Feb;166(2):454–5.

Miteva M, Tosti A. 'A detective look' at hair biopsies from African American patients. Br J Dermatol. 2012 Jun; 166(6):1289–94.

Pincus LB, Price VH, McCalmont TH. The amount counts: distinguishing neutrophil-mediated and lymphocyte-mediated cicatricial alopecia by compound follicles. J Cutan Pathol. 2011;38(1):1–4.

Quaresma MV, Mariño Alvarez AM, Miteva M. Dermatoscopic-pathologic correlation of lichen simplex chronicus on the scalp: 'broom fibres, gear wheels and hamburgers'. J Eur Acad Dermatol Venereol. 2016 Feb;30(2):343–5.

Royer MC, Sperling LC. Splitting hairs: the 'hamburger sign' in trichotillomania. J Cutan Pathol. Sep 2006;33 Suppl 2:63–64.

Saceda-Corralo D, Nusbaum AG, Romanelli P, Miteva M. A case of circumscribed scalp morphea with perineural lymphocytes on pathology. Skin Appendage Disord. 2017 Oct;3(4):175–8. doi: 10.1159/000471855. Epub 2017 Apr 29

Thibaut S, Gaillard O, Bouhanna P, Cannell DW, Bernard BA. Human hair shape is programmed from the bulb. Br J Dermatol. 2005 Apr;152(4):632–8.

Pitfalls in Pathologic Diagnosis of Hair Disorders

7

In the middle of difficulty lies opportunity.
Albert Einstein

Contents

GENERAL CONCEPTS

The most common pitfalls or difficulties in scalp biopsies for hair loss arise from the facts that:

1. Many hair disorders have insidious onset and therefore clinico-pathological correlation may fail at the time of the histologic diagnosis; in subtle cases, trichoscopy may help. (*Example*: identifying individual terminal hairs with subtle peripilar casts in the frontal hairline in women with otherwise preserved vellus hairs helps to diagnose early frontal fibrosing alopecia, FFA).
2. Most hair loss conditions do not have specific features and therefore stratifying the clinical and histologic diagnosis in cases with overlapping features may be difficult (*Example*: cases of folliculitis decalvans and lichen planopilaris phenotypic spectrum, FDLPPPS).
3. Patients can have more than one hair loss diagnosis at the same time (*Example*: lichen planopilaris (LPP) in patients with androgenetic alopecia (AGA) or trichotillomania in children with concomitant alopecia areata).
4. There is a common follicular "response" to inflammation/injury in different hair disorders (*Example*: abrupt onset of telogen shift in pressure-induced alopecia, trichotillomania and alopecia areata).
5. Suboptimal quality of the specimen (*Example*: a 2 mm specimen obtained from an area with lost follicular openings in a patient with active scarring alopecia or a 2 mm specimen obtained from a patient with diffuse hair loss bisected on vertical sections).

MOST COMMON PITFALLS

1. LPP is overdiagnosed in biopsies from AGA.
   This problem has two common scenarios and one caveat:
   - Mild lymphocytic infiltrate and mild fibroplasia at the upper follicular level in AGA should not be overcalled LPP.

Dr. Whiting's fundamental work on hair counts in biopsies from male pattern AGA (J Am Acad Dermatol 1993; 28:755) showed that 64% of the biopsies revealed no or mild inflammation and/or fibrosis. *Mild inflammation* was considered a normal finding as it was present in same number among controls. *Moderate inflammation/fibrosis* was found in 36% (versus only 9% of the controls). The inflammatory infiltrate was composed mainly of lymphocytes and histiocytes and the perifollicular fibrosis was characterized as generally mild, consisting of loose, concentric layers of fibrotic collagen. He referred to the specimens without inflammation or with mild inflammation as *plain male pattern AGA* and the ones with significant inflammation/fibrosis as *complicated male pattern AGA* and showed that only 55% of the complicated cases had regrowth versus 77% of the plain cases without inflammation.

Researchers have found that follicular miniaturization is associated with a 2–2.5 times enlargement of the follicular dermal sheath (connective tissue sheath) composed of densely packed collagen bundles. It is considered that testosterone induces

TGF-β 1 and type I procollagen expression, which may contribute to the development of the perifollicular fibrosis in AGA. Li et al. recently discovered that fibrosis-related genes were overexpressed in the bugle portion of AGA-affected hair follicles implying that fibrosis participates in the disturbance of bulge stem cell conversion and leads to follicular miniaturization. This raises the question whether AGA and fibrosing alopecia in a pattern distribution (FAPD) represent actually a continuum?

Clues that can help distinguish the perifollicular inflammation and fibrosis at the upper follicular level (upper isthmus and infundibulum) in AGA from the lichenoid inflammation and fibrosis in LPP:

- The inflammation and the fibrosis in AGA are usually focal (affect individual follicles/follicular units) and restricted to the level of the isthmus and infundibulum (Figure 7.1), and the follicular architecture is preserved. The fibrosis can be called *fibroplasia* in the pathology report in order to help the clinician understand that this finding goes along with the follicular miniaturization, and is not a feature for scarring alopecia.
- The fibroplasia is composed of fine collagen bundles that appear as expanded connective tissue sheath. The perifollicular fibrosis in scarring alopecia is defined as concentric ("onion skin-like") lamellar fibrosis surrounding a zone of epithelial atrophy and is usually associated with clefts (Figure 7.2). Gomori trichrome stain can be helpful to distinguish ambiguous cases as the stain highlights the perifollicular collagen bundles of the connective tissue sheath, which in LPP usually remain separated from the follicular epithelium by a zone of concentric pale fibrosis (Figure 7.3).

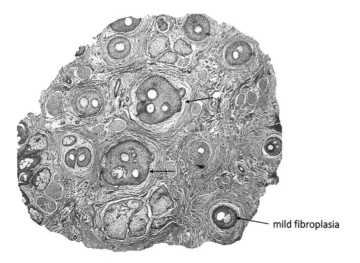

FIGURE 7.1 Mild perifollicular inflammation and fibroplasia (arrows) at the upper follicular level in AGA. Note that individual follicles or follicular units are affected.

- The outer root sheath of the affected follicles in AGA is preserved whereas in LPP there is consumption of the follicular epithelium (epithelial atrophy) (see Figures 7.2 and 7.4).
- Focal atrichia (follicular dropout) in AGA should not be overcalled LPP.

Follicular dropout may occur in longstanding nonscarring alopecia such as AGA due to the persistence of increased number of non-cycling, usually avascular fibrous streamers (FS) (Figures 7.5 and 7.6). The focal atrichia is associated with significantly decreased follicular counts, terminal:vellus ratio and number of follicles/mm². There is no lichenoid inflammation and perifollicular fibrosis and the sebaceous glands are intact.

It should be remembered that in horizontal sections at the level of the reticular dermis the perifollicular vascular plexus of the fibrous streamer disappears so that it looks like whorled delicate collagen (see Figure 7.5). Therefore, the viability of the FS based on its vascularity should be assessed at the level of the lower dermis and subdermis: viable FS show many small blood vessels and remnants of trichilemmal gray vitreous membrane versus more homogenized crumpled degenerate elastic material (Arao Perkins bodies) in non-cycling streamers (Figure 7.7). To establish if the focal areas of follicular dropout are follicular scars or avascular FS, polarized light microscopy can be used as human collagen is known to be birefringent on polarization and therefore follicular scars polarize whereas FS do not (Figure 7.8).

Elastic stain (elastic Verhoeff-Van Gieson, EVG) has also been reported helpful in distinguishing follicular scars from FS based on the pattern of the elastic network (intact elastic network composed of delicate and thin elastic without elastic network attenuation, loss, clumping, thickening or recoil versus central attenuation and loss of the elastic network with peripheral clumping and recoil of elastic fibers in follicular scars).

- *Caveat:* Early/focal/subtle LPP may co-exist with AGA: in fact, unrecognized LPP in the AGA area can be a pitfall for hair transplantation. Patients usually present with subtle erythema and scaling co-localized in the area of patterned thinning without well-formed patches. They may be treated for seborrheic dermatitis for years. Trichoscopy can be of significant help as it identifies small tufts of 2–4 hairs emerging from the same ostium surrounded by erythema, peripilar casts, and associated with hair thinning. This is the optimal site for the trichoscopy-guided biopsy (Figure 7.9). Histology should be performed on horizontal sections as many times only a portion of the follicles are affected. There are classic findings for LPP consisting of usually focal follicular dropout, individual or compound follicles

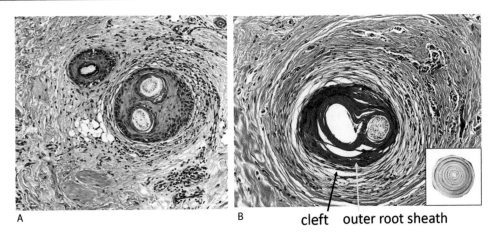

cleft   outer root sheath

FIGURE 7.2 In AGA (A), the fibrosis is less organized in layers and the outer root sheath is intact compared to scarring alopecia (lichen planopilaris in B): note the layered fibrosis in an onion-skin pattern (inset) and the atrophy of the outer root sheath in LPP.

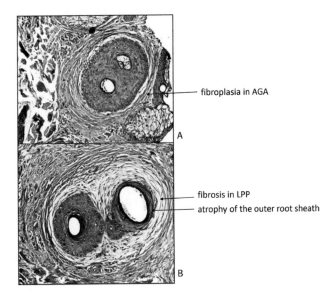

fibroplasia in AGA

fibrosis in LPP
atrophy of the outer root sheath

FIGURE 7.3 (A) Gomori trichrome stain highlights the perifollicular fibroplasia in AGA as blue fine collagen fibers surrounding intact follicular epithelium. (B) In LPP, the pale zone of concentric perifollicular fibrosis remains unstained and there is atrophy of the follicular epithelium.

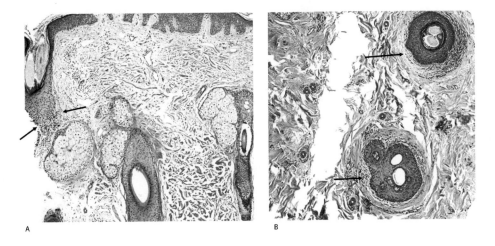

FIGURE 7.4 Examples of two different cases of AGA misdiagnosed as LPP due to the presence of infundibular inflammation and fibroplasia (arrows). Note the intact follicular epithelium and preservation of the sebaceous glands (on A). In such cases, I would recommend to my patients to use a topical steroid to address the inflammatory and fibrotic component.

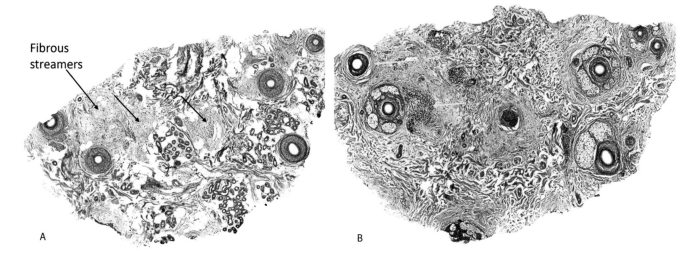

Fibrous streamers

FIGURE 7.5   (A) A case of advanced AGA with focal atrichia shows on pathology areas of follicular dropout due to non-cycling avascular fibrous streamers with elastic globules. (B) The same case shows mild inflammation and fibroplasia at the infundibular level (yellow arrows).

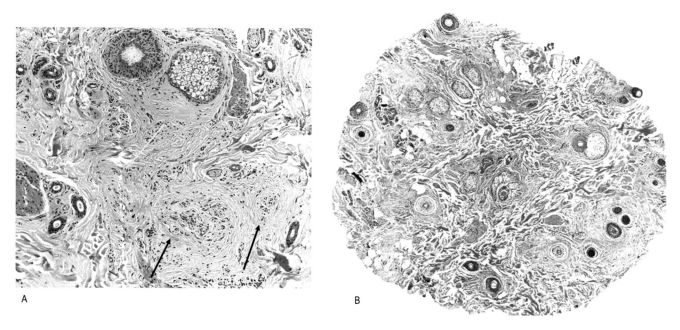

FIGURE 7.6   (A) Two other cases of advanced AGA with focal atrichia demonstrate follicular dropout due to non-cycling fibrous streamers aggregated in the lower dermis (black arrows). Note the significantly decreased follicular density (18 follicles) and the presence of avascular FS (yellow arrows) in the dermis (B).

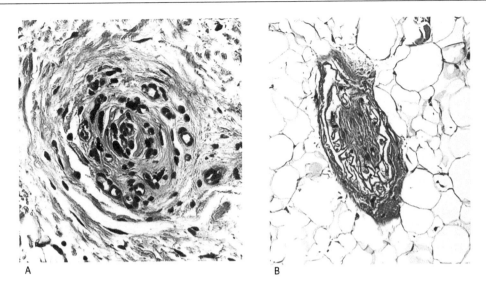

FIGURE 7.7   A viable FS with pronounced vascularity in (A) alopecia areata and hyalinized FS with decreased vascularity and bluish convoluted elastic material in AGA (B).

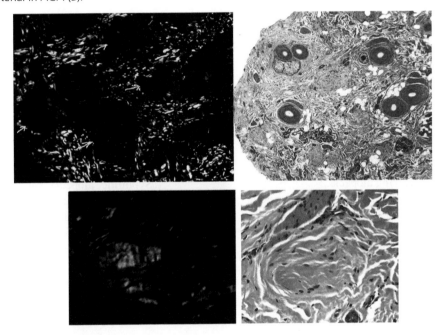

FIGURE 7.8   FS do not polarize (upper row of images) versus true follicular scars (low row).

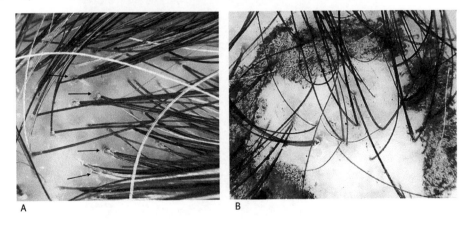

FIGURE 7.9   (A, B) Optimal sites for a biopsy in two patients with clinical features for patterned thinning but trichoscopic features for LPP show groups of 2–4 hairs emerging as one stem from a single ostium in the same area. Note also the peripilar casts (×10).

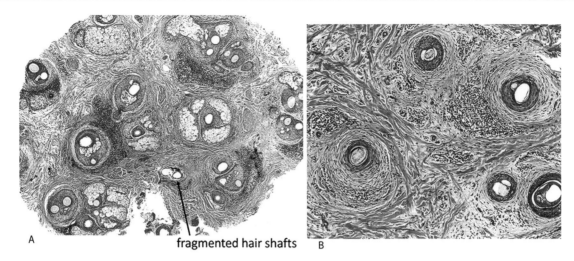

A   fragmented hair shafts   B

FIGURE 7.10 (A, B) Cases of focal LPP co-localized to the area of patterned thinning in AGA. Note the perifollicular fibrosis and lichenoid inflammation, together with follicular atrophy at the upper isthmus level.

with perifollicular fibrosis and lichenoid inflammation (Figure 7.10). The clinician should proceed with trichoscopy-guided scalp biopsies. In such cases, two biopsies may be more helpful to avoid error and to assess the extent of the involvement. Once diagnosed and started on treatment, in my experience these patients may have better prognosis versus those with classic LPP.

2. Absence of sebaceous glands in elderly patients may be misleading for scarring alopecia.

Atrophy of the sebaceous glands is a feature of menopause/adrenopause and therefore scalp biopsy from elderly patients has decreased number and size of sebaceous glands. Sebaceous gland loss is a common early finding among scarring alopecia that is even considered pathogenic; however, it is associated with other features such as inflammation involving the sebaceous glands, including the sebaceous ducts, perifollicular fibrosis and lichenoid inflammation (Figure 7.11).

3. "Swarm of bees" bulbar infiltrate *is not specific* for alopecia areata.

The inflammatory infiltrate in LPP may extend deep in dermis and even into the subdermis where the bulbs of the follicles reside (Figure 7.12).

Syphilitic alopecia can be indistinguishable from alopecia areata: helpful clues include plasma cells in the FS and in perivascular distribution (Figure 7.13). Herpes zoster infection in the scalp has been associated with hair loss mimicking alopecia areata patches and shows similar peribulbar swarm of bees infiltrate on histology (Figure 7.14).

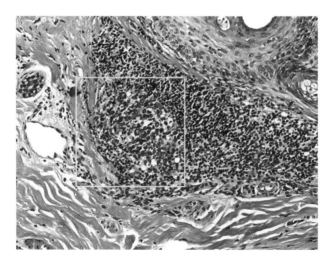

FIGURE 7.11 Lichenoid inflammation involving the sebaceous lobule at the level of the isthmus in LPP.

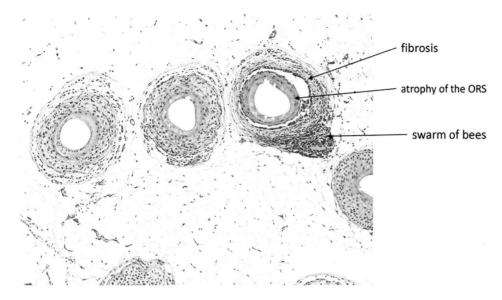

FIGURE 7.12   Swarm of bees-like infiltrate in the subdermis in LPP. The infiltrate is suprabulbar; there is also perifollicular fibrosis and atrophy of the outer root sheath (ORS).

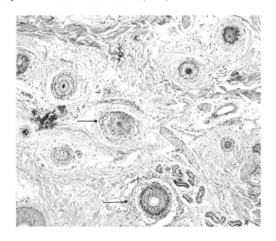

FIGURE 7.13   Swarm of bees-like infiltrate in syphilitic alopecia.

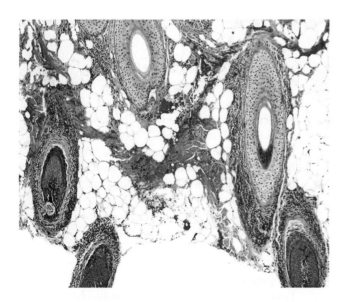

FIGURE 7.14   Swarm of bees-like infiltrate in a case of herpes zoster involving the scalp.

FURTHER READING

Al-Zaid T, Vanderweil S, Zembowicz A, Lyle S. Sebaceous gland loss and inflammation in scarring alopecia: a potential role in pathogenesis. J Am Acad Dermatol. 2011 Sep;65(3):597–603.

Baquerizo Nole KL, Nusbaum B, Pinto GM, Miteva M. Lichen planopilaris in the androgenetic alopecia area: a pitfall for hair transplantation. Skin Appendage Disord. 2015 Mar;1(1):49–53.

Jaworsky C, Kligman AM, Murphy GF. Characterization of inflammatory infiltrates in male pattern alopecia: implications for pathogenesis. Br J Dermatol. 1992 Sep;127(3):239–46.

Miteva M, Tosti A. Polarized microscopy as a helpful tool to distinguishchronic nonscarring alopecia from scarring alopecia. Arch Dermatol. 2012 Jan;148(1):91–4.

Sperling LC. Scarring alopecia and the dermatopathologist. J Cutan Pathol. Aug 2001;28(7):333–42.

Tan T, Guitart J, Gerami P, Yazdan P. Elastic staining in differentiating between follicular streamers and follicular scars in horizontal scalp biopsy sections. Am J Dermatopathol. 2018 Apr;40(4):254–8.

Wong D, Goldberg LJ. The depth of inflammation in frontal fibrosing alopecia and lichen planopilaris: a potential distinguishing feature. J Am Acad Dermatol. 2017 Jun;76(6):1183–4.

Yoo HG, Kim JS, Lee SR, Pyo HK, Moon HI, Lee JH, Kwon OS, Chung JH, Kim KH, Eun HC, Cho KH. Perifollicular fibrosis: pathogenetic role in androgenetic alopecia. Biol Pharm Bull. 2006 Jun;29(6):1246–50.

Li K, Liu F, Sun Y, Gan Y, Zhu D, Wang H, Qu Q, Wang J, Chen R, Fan Z, Liu B, Fu D, Miao Y, Hu Z. Association of fibrosis in the bulge portion with hair follicle miniaturization in androgenetic alopecia. J Am Acad Dermatol. 2021 Feb 2:S0190–9622(21)00238–3.

Alopecia Areata

8

Contents

GENERAL CONCEPTS

- Alopecia areata (AA) presents as hair loss in patches. It is an autoimmune phenomenon resulting from disturbance in the hair follicle immune privilege (IP) that leads to anagen inhibition. IP is an evolutionary adaptation to protect vital structures (such as the central nervous system, the anterior chamber of the eye, the testes and the placenta) from the potentially damaging effects of an inflammatory immune response. The bulge throughout the hair cycle and the *bulb in anagen* are immune privileged. On the one side, the matrix cells do not express major histocompatibility complex I (MHC I) antigens and, on the other side, there is a local production of potent immunosuppressive molecules such as α-MSH and TGF-β1, which protect the IP. A breakthrough in the immune shield mediated by INF-gamma expression leads to recruitment of activated CD4 T cells and CD8+ NKG2D+ effector memory T cells in the peribulbar area of the anagen follicle ("swarm of bees" infiltrate).
- The anagen inhibition results in tapered off hair shafts – dystrophic hairs and miniaturized hairs (sometimes, the follicles may miniaturize for 1–2 cycles or even persist as *nanogen* follicles without visible regrowth [see below]).

- AA's course is characterized by 3 stages: acute, subacute and chronic (Figure 8.1). There is also a recovery stage, which is rarely biopsied.
- The histopathologic features of alopecia areata depend on the stage of the current episode as described by David Whiting in his fundamental work *Histopathologic Features of Alopecia Areata: A New Look*.

MAIN HISTOLOGIC FEATURES

Acute Stage (1–3 Months)

- On histology, the follicular density is generally preserved. On trichoscopy, the hair morphology is altered by cadaverized (black dots) and broken hairs (Figure 8.2). Terminal pigmented shafts of inflamed follicles abruptly become weak resulting into hair breakage at different levels and clumps of amorphous pigmented material in the follicular ostia.
- Peribulbar lymphocytic infiltrate (known as "the swarm of bees") around terminal follicles (both anagen and catagen follicles) in early episodes and around vellus follicles in repeated episodes (Figure 8.3). The infiltrate invades the matrix and the follicular epithelium (Figure 8.4). Lymphocytes can also be detected in the fibrous streamers, together with eosinophils and pigmented casts (Figure 8.5).

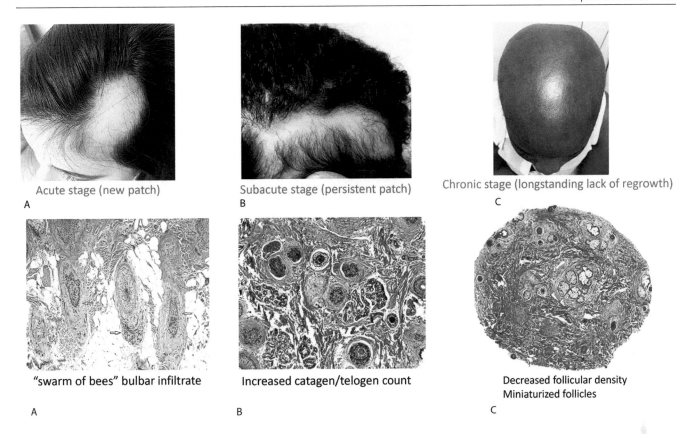

Acute stage (new patch)

A

Subacute stage (persistent patch)

B

Chronic stage (longstanding lack of regrowth)

C

"swarm of bees" bulbar infiltrate

A

Increased catagen/telogen count

B

Decreased follicular density
Miniaturized follicles

C

FIGURE 8.1   The clinical stages of AA with histologic correlation: (A) Acute stage (new patch) with corresponding "swarm of bees" bulbar infiltrate; (B) subacute stage (persitent patch) with corresponding increased catagen/telogen count; (C) chronic stage (longstanding lack of regrowth) with corresponding decreased follicular density and miniaturize follicles.

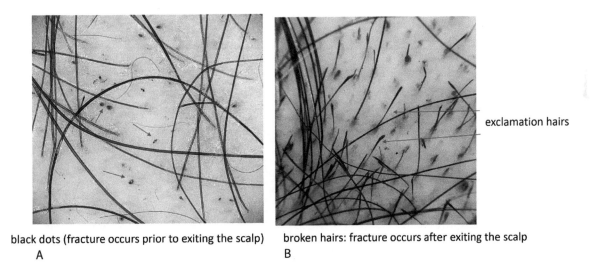

exclamation hairs

black dots (fracture occurs prior to exiting the scalp)

A

broken hairs: fracture occurs after exiting the scalp

B

FIGURE 8.2   (A) Black dots, also known as cadaverized hairs (the fracture occurs prior to exiting the scalp) (×20) and (B) exclamation hairs (fracture occurs after exiting the scalp) (×10) are variants of dystrophic hairs and correspond to inflamed terminal catagen/telogen follicles and amorphous pigmented material in the follicular ostia.

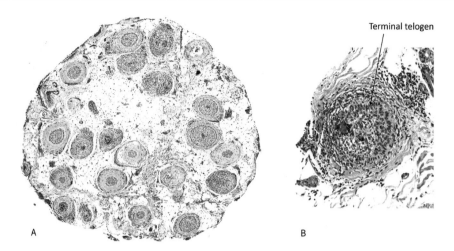

FIGURE 8.3   Dense inflammatory bulbar infiltrates (swarm of bees) in alopecia areata.

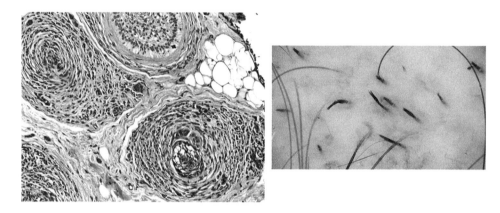

FIGURE 8.4   (A) The swarm of bees infiltrate invades the follicular matrix which leads to abrupt catagen/telogen shift, weakening of the hair shaft and hair breakage (B) (×40).

Caveat: The swarm of bees infiltrate is not specific for AA and can be detected also in other conditions (see Chapter 7). It is also not sensitive for the diagnosis as it is present only in the early stage of the disease.

- Increased number of catagen/telogen follicles (usually more than 50% and sometimes up to 90%) due to anagen "escape" of the affected follicles into catagen/telogen (Figure 8.6). The dystrophic hairs observed on trichoscopy are in fact catagen/telogen follicles (see Figure 8.4).
- Pigmented casts as coarse amorphous clumps of melanin in the fibrous streamers and within the infundibular ostia (Figure 8.7).
- Trichomalacia (incompletely keratinized, soft and distorted hair shafts) (Figure 8.8).
- *Nanogen* follicles can be found at any stage. According to David Whiting, they are diseased miniaturized follicles that are difficult to categorize as anagen, catagen or telogen. They have a thinner epithelial matrix, inner and outer root sheaths and are detected in the mid and upper dermis because they cycle faster.

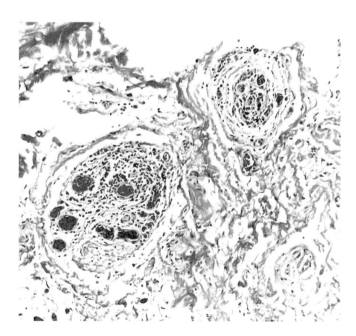

FIGURE 8.5   Fibrous streamers with lymphocytes and pigmented casts in AA.

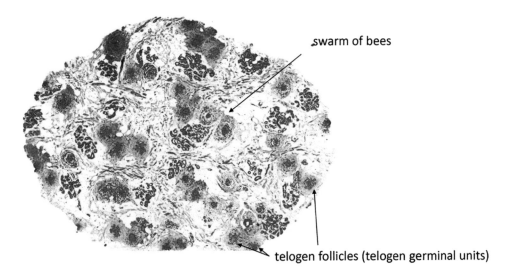

FIGURE 8.6 In this example of acute stage AA, virtually all follicles are in catagen/telogen phase and there is swarm of bees inflammation.

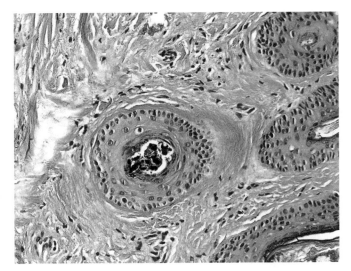

FIGURE 8.7 Pigmented casts in an infundibular ostium in AA.

Nanogen follicles may show remnants of pink inner root sheath but usually none or pencil-like thin hair shaft (Figure 8.9). In the histologic report, they should be mentioned separately in the follicular counts.

Subacute Stage (3–12 Months)

- There could be decreased follicular density with less dystrophic hairs on trichoscopy
- An increased number of catagen/telogen follicles (catagen, telogen and telogen germinal units are counted together) (Figure 8.10)
- Inflammatory cells such as lymphocytes, eosinophils and mast cells together with pigmented casts may persist in the fibrous streamers

Chronic/Longstanding Stage (12 Months Onward)

- A decreased number of terminal follicles, which corresponds on trichoscopy to yellow dots, non-visible follicular openings and/or vellus hairs (Figure 8.11).
- A increased number of miniaturized follicles with significantly decreased terminal:vellus ratio of average 1.3:1 (Figure 8.12).

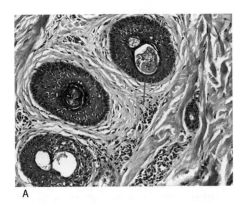
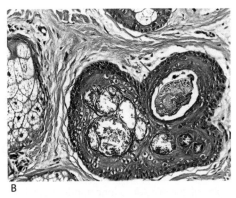

FIGURE 8.8 (A, B) Examples of trichomalacia (arrows) in the follicular ostia in AA.

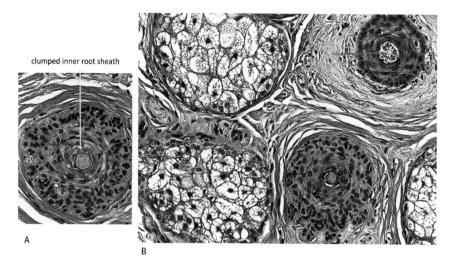

FIGURE 8.9 Nanogen follicles are small follicles of mixed phenotype: it is hard to categorize them as anagen, catagen or telogen. They usually have none a clumped inner root sheath (A, yellow arrow), none or very thin non-keratinized hair shaft (B, blue arrow).

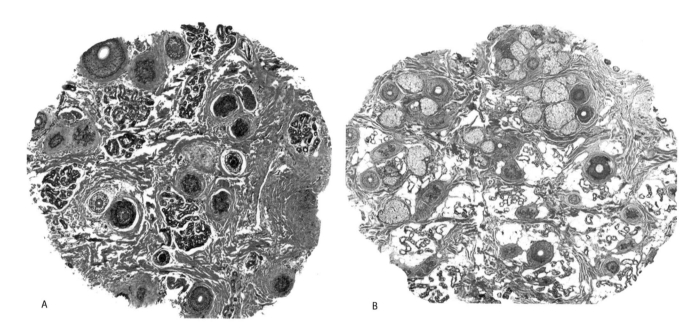

FIGURE 8.10 Examples of subacute stage AA with increased telogen count of 56% (A) and 78% (B).

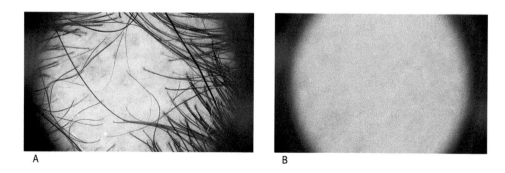

FIGURE 8.11 Examples of chronic AA: a longstanding patch without regrowth shows yellow dots (A, ×20) and alopecia universalis with non-visible follicular ostia (B, ×20).

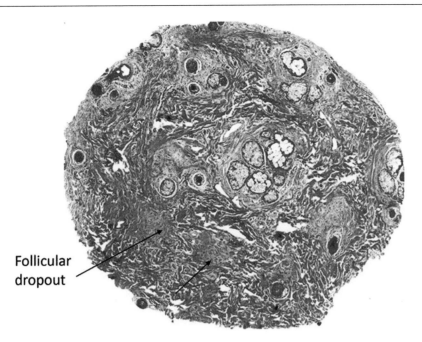

Follicular
dropout

FIGURE 8.12 In this longstanding case of alopecia universalis, there are 13 vellus follicles which make total density of 1 follicle/mm². The chance of regrowth is borderline to poor. The differential diagnosis from traction alopecia is difficult without clinical information.

- This stage may resemble longstanding androgenetic alopecia or even traction alopecia due to areas of follicular dropout (Figure 8.13).
- There is usually no inflammation or mild inflammatory infiltrate can be noted around the bulbs of the miniaturized follicles in the upper dermis as in the reactivation stage.

- Less than 1 follicle/mm² in this stage is considered as little likelihood for regrowth considering that the normal follicular density is 2–3.1 follicles/mm² (a 4 mm punch biopsy has circumference of 12.6 mm² and a 3 mm punch biopsy has 7 mm²).

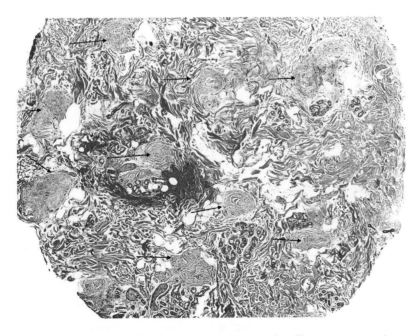

FIGURE 8.13 More examples of alopecia universalis: there are many non-cycling fibrous streamers (arrows) but no follicles.

Recovery Stage

- Increasing numbers of terminal anagen follicles from regrowth of miniaturized follicles (Figure 8.14)

PEARLS

- Early discoid lupus erythematosus may mimic AA (Figure 8.15) – look for interface dermatitis and perieccrine inflammatory infiltrate.

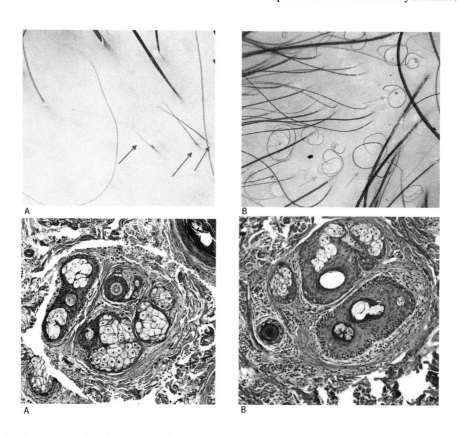

FIGURE 8.14   Upright short regrowing hairs (A) and pigtail hairs (B) correspond to vellus follicles and intermediate size terminal anagen follicles.

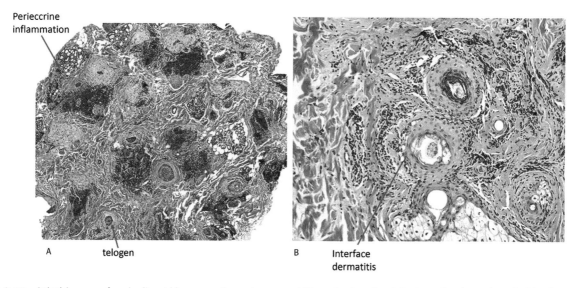

FIGURE 8.15   (A) This case of early discoid lupus erythematosus could be mistaken for AA given the dense lymphoid inflammation at the bulbar level and increased telogen count. However, note that the infiltrate is not strictly follicular; it is also perivascular and perieccrine (B). There is also interface vacuolar damage of the follicular epithelium at the isthmus level.

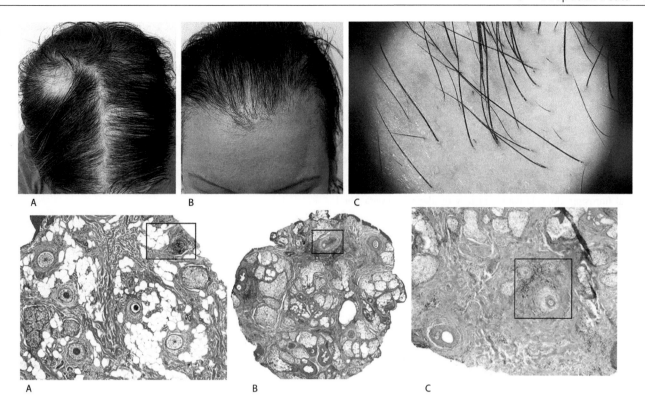

FIGURE 8.16 (A) This patient has a patch and a long history of AA. She noticed reduced hairline recently (B). Trichoscopy shows absence of vellus hairs, loss of follicular openings, broken hairs and short regrowing hairs (×20). Biopsy from the hairline shows mixed features for AA (swarm of bees infiltrate and follicular miniaturization) (A) but also perifollicular fibrosis and lichenoid infiltrate at the infundibular level (B, C). This association has been reported by us and others.

- Syphilitic alopecia may mimic acute stage AA (look for plasma cells and perivascular infiltrate with endothelial swelling); pressure-induced alopecia and trichotillomania may mimic subacute stage AA – look for coarse, abnormal bizarre-shaped pigmented casts and prominent trichomalacia (hamburger sign, zip and button sign), and absence of miniaturized follicles including nanogen follicles.

- Co-existence of AA with other hair disorders such as trichotillomania or frontal fibrosing alopecia is possible (Figure 8.16).
- Lipoatrophy due to steroid injections presents as downsized fat lobules, smaller fat cells and an increased number of capillaries (Figure 8.17).

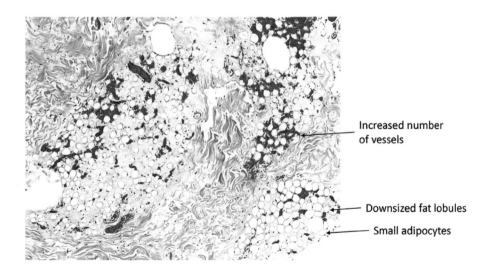

Increased number of vessels

Downsized fat lobules

Small adipocytes

FIGURE 8.17 Cutaneous lipoatrophy in AA injected continuously with intralesional steroids.

FURTHER READING

Chung HJ, Goldberg LJ. Histologic features of chronic cutaneous lupus erythematosus of the scalp using horizontal sectioning: emphasis on follicular findings. J Am Acad Dermatol. 2017 Aug;77(2):349–55.

Dy LC, Whiting DA. Histopathology of alopecia areata, acute and chronic: why is it important to the clinician? Dermatol Ther. 2011 May–Jun;24(3):369–74.

Lin J, Zikry J, Atanaskova-Mesinkovska N. Development of frontal fibrosing alopecia with a history of alopecia areata. Int J Trichology. 2018 Jan–Feb;10(1):29–30.

Paus R, Ito N, Takigawa M, Ito T. The hair follicle and immune privilege. J Investig Dermatol Symp Proc. 2003 Oct;8(2):188–94.

Peckham SJ, Sloan SB, Elston DM. Histologic features of alopecia areata other than peribulbar lymphocytic infiltrates. J Am Acad Dermatol. 2011 Sep;65(3):615–20.

Rajabi F, Drake LA, Senna MM, Rezaei N. Alopecia areata: a review of disease pathogenesis. Br J Dermatol. 2018 Nov;179(5):1033–48.

Whiting DA. Histopathologic features of alopecia areata: a new look. Arch Dermatol. 2003 Dec;139(12):1555–9.

Alopecia Areata Incognita

9

Contents

GENERAL CONCEPTS

Alopecia areata incognito or Alopecia areata incognita (AAI) is a diffuse alopecia characterized by acute hair shedding leading to pronounced hair thinning of the whole scalp in women without clinical and laboratory findings that suggest acute telogen effluvium.

- *Clinical examination* shows diffusely reduced hair density, which may be more pronounced on the androgen dependent scalp (Figure 9.1). The pull test is positive for telogen roots at different degrees of maturation with a high prevalence of early telogen roots, characterized by presence of the epithelial envelope surrounding the club hair (Figure 9.2).
- *Trichoscopy* shows yellow dots and short regrowing hairs. Dystrophic hairs, typical for diffuse alopecia areata, are absent (Figure 9.3).
- The prognosis is usually favorable with rapid response to steroid treatment (see Figure 9.1).
- In classic AA, alopecic patches are formed because there are localized groups of hairs in the early anagen stage (with high mitotic activity) that are most vulnerable to immune disruption and undergo simultaneously anagen inhibition. According to Alfredo Rebora, AAI is more common in patients with androgenetic alopecia because shortening of the hair cycle reduces the number of follicles with high mitotic activity and increases the number of follicles with low mitotic activity that shift to telogen instead of becoming dystrophic. In AAI, the hair loss is therefore diffuse and telogenic.

MAIN HISTOLOGIC FEATURES

- The diagnosis requires horizontal sections for follicular counts and ratios.
- Preserved number or follicular units and decreased number of terminal follicles (Table 9.1).
- Decreased terminal: vellus ratio, an average ratio of 3.3: 1 (normal ratio is ≥4:1) (Figure 9.4)
- Increased number of follicles in catagen and telogen stages (mean count of 37%) instead of the normal count of up to 15% (Figure 9.5).
- Presence of increased number of telogen germinal units, and/or small basaloid aggregates of cells with round, irregular or polygonal shape, lack of hair shaft and no apoptosis in the outer root sheath, referred to as "small telogen follicles" (Figures 9.6 and 9.7). These are telogen follicles bisected just above the level of the vestigial hair bulb and below the level of the cornified club. These "small telogen follicles" are most likely miniaturized telogen follicles related to the nanogen follicles described in AA. They should be mentioned in the report and counted towards the vellus follicles.
- Dilated infundibular openings (measuring: 0.02–0.05 mm versus normal diameter of 0.01 mm) (Figure 9.8).

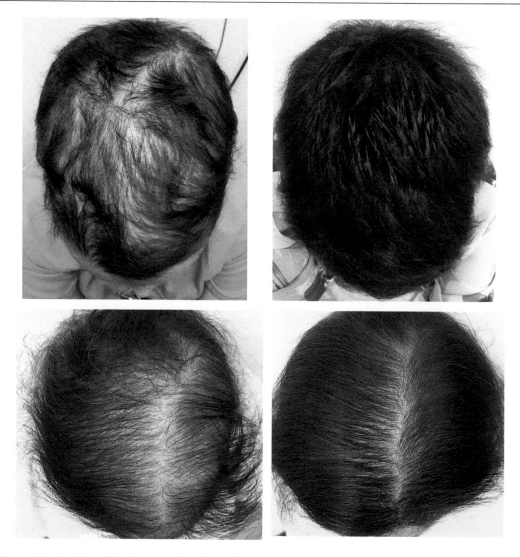

FIGURE 9.1   Two patients with AAI (before and after 3 months of treatment with topical minoxidil and topical steroid).

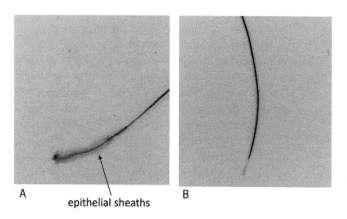

A   epithelial sheaths   B

FIGURE 9.2   (A) Early telogen hair from AAI and (B) a telogen club hair for comparison.

FURTHER READING

Miteva M, Misciali C, Fanti PA, Tosti A. Histopathologic features of alopecia areata incognito: a review of 46 cases. J Cutan Pathol. 2012 Jun;39(6):596–602.

Rebora A. Alopecia areata incognita. J Am Acad Dermatol. 2011 Dec;65(6):1228.

Rebora A. Alopecia areata incognita: a comment. Clinics (Sao Paulo). 2011;66(8):1481–2.

Tosti A, Whiting D, Iorizzo M, Pazzaglia M, Misciali C, Vincenzi C, Micali G. The role of scalp dermoscopy in the diagnosis of alopecia areata incognita. J Am Acad Dermatol. 2008 Jul;59(1):64–7.

Whiting DA. Chronic telogen effluvium: increased scalp hair shedding in middle-aged women. J Am Acad Dermatol. Dec 1996;35(6):899–906

Whiting DA. Diagnostic and predictive value of horizontal sections of scalp biopsy specimens in male pattern androgenetic alopecia. J Am Acad Dermatol. May 1993;28(5 Pt 1):755–763.

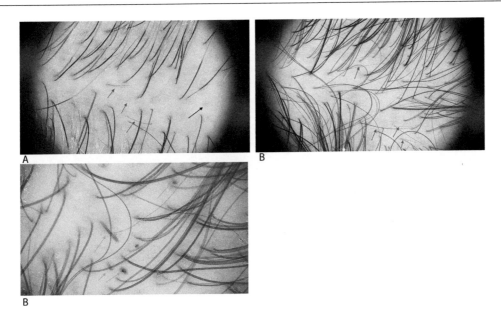

FIGURE 9.3 Yellow dots (black arrow) and regrowing hairs (red arrows) in a patient with AAI (before (A) and after treatment (B)). Dystrophic hairs (blue arrows) in a patient with diffuse AA (C).

TABLE 9.1 Comparative follicular counts and ratios in AAI versus normal scalp and versus other common forms of non-scarring diffuse alopecia in women

FOLLICULAR VARIABLES	NORMAL SCALP	AAI	CHRONIC TELOGEN EFFLUVIUM	ANDROGENETIC ALOPECIA
Follicular units	13	10	13	13
Terminal follicles	35	17	35	23
Vellus/Miniaturized follicles	5	8	4	12
Fibrous streamers	1-2	6	3	8
Anagen: Telogen ratio (%)	93.5:6.5	63:37	89:11	83.2:16.8
Terminal: Vellus ratio	7:1	3:1	9:1	1.9:1

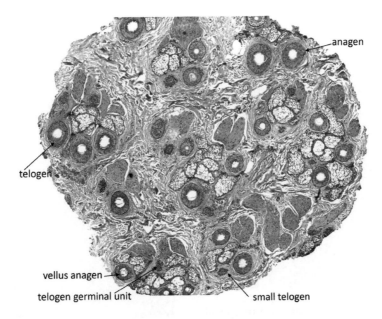

FIGURE 9.4 AAI in a patient with AGA: there are 32 follicles (10 terminal anagen, 4 terminal telogen, 7 vellus anagen and 11 "small telogen/telogen germinal units". The terminal:vellus ratio is 0.8:1 and the telogen count is 29%.

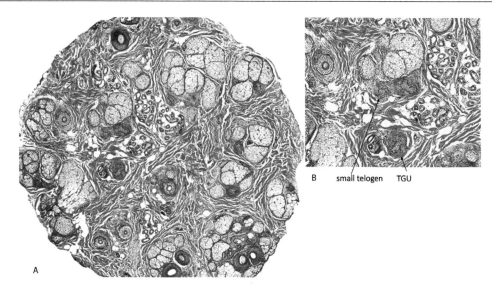

FIGURE 9.5   (A, B) Another case of AAI: note the low follicular density and the increased number of telogen follicles including small telogen follicles and TGUs.

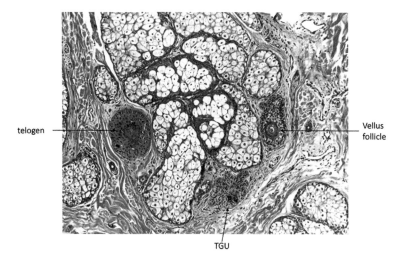

FIGURE 9.6   This follicular unit "embodies the hallmark" of AAI: constellation of miniaturization with increased telogen count (including small telogen follicles and/or TGUs).

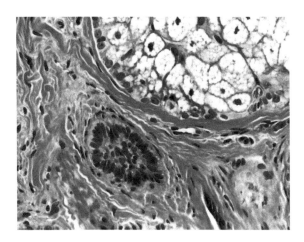

FIGURE 9.7   Example of a basaloid aggregate of a polygonal shape that represents a small telogen follicle. Note the absence of a hair shaft and apoptosis.

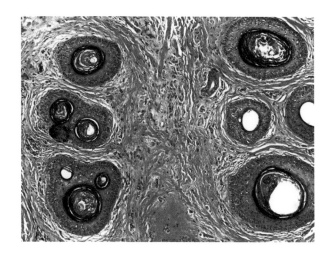

FIGURE 9.8   Dilated infundibula in AAI.

Telogen Effluvium

10

Contents

GENERAL CONCEPTS

- Telogen effluvium (TE) was first described as diffuse cyclic hair loss in women in whom "systemic stresses, disease, or physiologic situations cause many scalp hairs to enter the resting phase prematurely".
- TE presents as acquired diffuse scalp shedding and thinning; it was originally classified by Headington into five categories and re-classified more recently by Rebora into three:
  - Premature teloptosis (premature hair dislodgement) such as after starting minoxidil treatment
  - Collective teloptosis (delayed anagen and telogen release) following synchronization of the hair cycle such as in neonatal TE, postpartum TE and hormonal-induced TE (estrogen and progesterone)
  - Premature entry in telogen (immediate anagen release due to premature interruption of the anagen phase and transition into telogen); dystrophic shedding occurs in follicles in early anagen (characterized by high mitotic activity), whereas acceleration to telogen occurs in follicles in late anagen phase; examples include drug-induced TE or dietary-induced TE
- Acute TE usually follows a childbirth, acute illness and lasts up to 6 months with full recovery of hair. It is therefore rarely biopsied.
- In chronic TE (CTE), the hair loss is persistent, diffuse and involves the entire scalp but can be difficult to appreciate as many patients present with full head of hair (Figure 10.1). There is most pronounced thinning of the bitemporal sides and the ponytail. It can last many months to years and can have a fluctuant course. Most biopsies are taken in this stage. Trichoscopy shows empty follicular ostia, upright regrowing hairs and lack of hair shaft variability (Figure 10.2).

  Caveat: Trichoscopy is not diagnostic in CTE; CTE and androgenetic alopecia (AGA) may co-exist in the same patient.

MAIN HISTOLOGIC FEATURES

- Biopsies from TE should be obtained from the parietal scalp since this is an androgen dependent area, which would help to exclude AGA. The biopsies should not be taken from the temporal scalp, as there is normally an increased number of short thin hairs. The biopsies should be processed for horizontal sections to provide follicular counts and ratios.
- Acute TE shows normal terminal:vellus ratio but increased telogen count up to 25%.
- Biopsies from CTE are *indistinguishable* from biopsies of normal scalp.
- There is none or slightly decreased follicular density with normal (≥4:1), and even increased terminal:vellus ratio of 9:1 (Figure 10.3). The telogen count is usually normal (up to 15%) or slightly increased in active phases of shedding as CTE has fluctuating course.

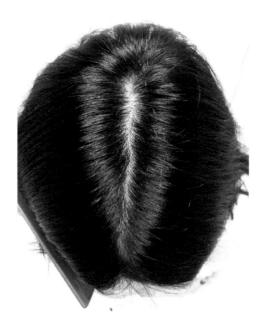

FIGURE 10.1 Chronic telogen effluvium: usually, there is no visibly reduced hair density.

- Mild inflammation and fibrosis is possible at the infundibular level in about 1/3 of the biopsies similar to control biopsies from normal scalp (Figure 10.4). Moderate inflammation and fibrosis are more common in AGA.

PEARLS

- Terminal telogen follicles (catagen, telogen and telogen germinal units) are counted towards the terminal follicles. Care should be taken not to count the same follicles several times based on their distinct morphologic features at the different levels (Figure 10.5).
- Vellus telogen follicles should be counted towards the vellus follicles, as they are miniaturized follicles (Figure 10.6). Careful examination of all levels including the infundibulum allows for tracking the vellus telogen follicles.

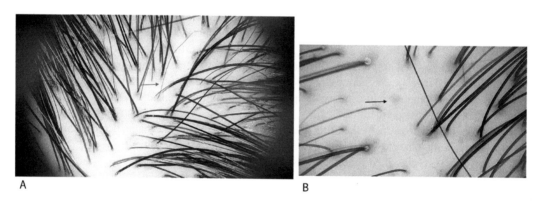

A   B

FIGURE 10.2 Trichoscopy shows no specific features. There is no hair shaft variability (A, ×20). There are regrowing hairs with tapered ends (A, red arrow) and empty dots (B, ×40, black arrow).

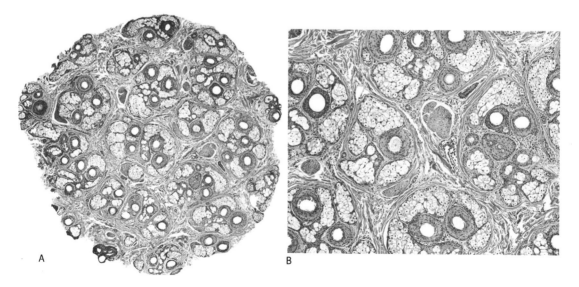

A   B

FIGURE 10.3 (A, B) CTE: the follicular density is 47 follicles. The terminal:vellus ratio is 7:1. The telogen count is 5%.

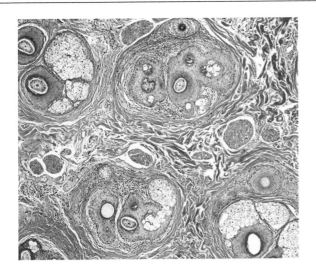

FIGURE 10.4 Mild perifollicular inflammation can be seen in chronic telogen effluvium as well as in the normal scalp.

FURTHER READING

Guy WB, Edmundson WF. Diffuse cyclic hair loss in women. Arch Dermatol. 1960 Feb;81:205–7.

Headington JT. Telogen effluvium. New concepts and review. Arch Dermatol. 1993 Mar;129(3):356–63.

Rebora A. Proposing a simpler classification of telogen effluvium. Skin Appendage Disord. 2016 Sep;2 (1-2):35–38. Epub 2016 May 18.

Whiting DA. Chronic telogen effluvium: increased scalp hair shedding in middle-aged women. J Am Acad Dermatol. 1996 Dec;35(6):899–906.

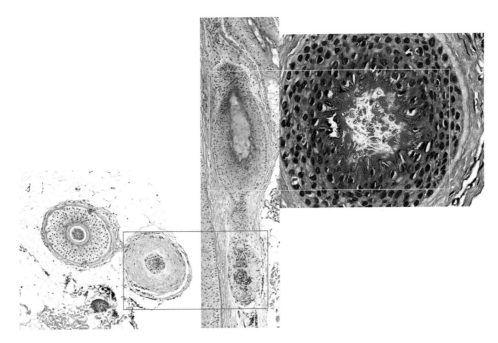

FIGURE 10.5 Telogen follicle at the level of the subdermis shows thickened vitreous layer (blue blox). At the level of the isthmus the club hair presents as degenerated serrated keratin mass (yellow box).

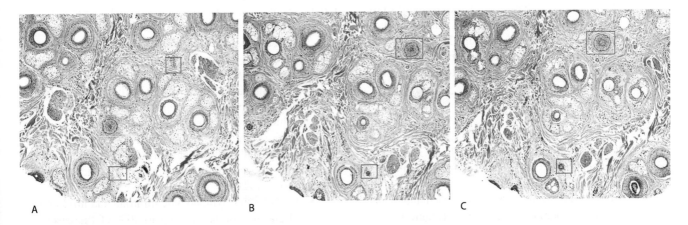

A   B   C

FIGURE 10.6 (A–C) Tracking the same vellus telogen follicles at step sections of the upper follicular level.

Androgenetic Alopecia

11

Contents

GENERAL CONCEPTS

Androgenetic alopecia (AGA) is an androgen-related hair disorder characterized by gradual and progressive, irreversible follicular miniaturization resulting in patterned (men and women) or diffuse (women) thinning in genetically predisposed individuals.

- This is the most common type of hair biopsy in the daily practice. Most biopsies are obtained from women.
- Men with classic AGA are rarely biopsied and a biopsy is usually done to exclude focal lichen planopilaris (LPP)/fibrosing alopecia in a pattern distribution (FAPD) (see also Chapter 7), especially prior to hair transplant surgery.
- Trichoscopy is very helpful for the diagnosis of AGA, which is based on detecting hair shaft variability. In women and men, usually 6 sites are studied in the parietal scalp. Two sites in the bitemporal scalp and one in the uninvolved occipital scalp can be added in men (for comparison) (Figure 11.1).
- Main trichoscopic features include:

  - Hair shaft variability (unisotrichosis): hair shafts of different thickness (thick, intermediate and vellus) with increased proportion of the vellus hairs (Figure 11.2)
  - Decreased number of hairs per follicular unit and increased number of single hairs (Figure 11.3)
  - Yellow dots (irregular distributed and mainly in frontal scalp) (Figure 11.4)
  - Peripilar sign (about 1 mm perifollicular brown halo corresponding to mild infundibular lymphocytic infiltrate and fine fibroplasia), which can be white in Fitzpatrick skin type IV-VI (Figure 11.5)

MAIN HISTOLOGIC FEATURES

There is an increased number of vellus follicles accounting for decreased terminal:vellus ratio (T:V) of less than 4:1 (Figure 11.6). As shown by Whiting, the average terminal:vellus ratio in 219 horizontally sectioned biopsies from women with AGA showed an average ratio of terminal to vellus hairs of 2.2:1. Mentioning the terminal:vellus ratio in the report helps to also guide the management as earlier cases (T:V ratio of 2.2–3.9) may require less complex management and have better prognosis.

- A common approach is to count the intermediate follicles together with the vellus follicles (see Chapter 4) (Figure 11.7).
- The vellus follicles should be counted at the isthmus level and above. Sometimes, only the very small dermal papilla of the vellus follicle is noted at the isthmus level in horizontal sections. Further step sections are required to visualize the entire vellus follicle and confirm the numbers (Figure 11.8).
- The telogen count may be slightly increased to about 19–20%.
- Perifollicular lymphocytic infiltrate and mild fibroplasia may be seen in up to 70% of the cases at

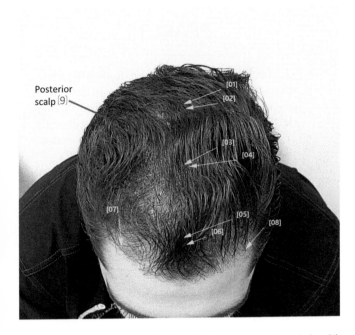

FIGURE 11.1 Posterior scalp (outside the patterned area) should be studied on trichoscopy for comparison.

the infundibular level, which can be overcalled as Lichen Planopilaris (see Chapter 7; Figure 11.9). Although AGA and FAPD may actually be considered a continuum and in some cases clear distinction is not possible, as a rule the perifollicular fibrosis in FAPD and LPP is concentrically layered and there is consumption of the follicular epithelium; there is more pronounced lichenoid infiltrate (Figure 11.10).

- Individual fragmented hair shafts can also be encountered in some biopsies of AGA, usually in longstanding/advanced AGA. Most likely, they are sequential to the rupture of those hair follicles showing lymphocytic inflammation and perifollicular fibroplasia (Figure 11.11). They can be seen also in FAPD.
- Advanced cases of AGA show focal atrichia (increased number of non-cycling fibrous streamers), which also can be mistaken for scarring alopecia (Figure 11.12).
- Using polarized light can help distinguish longstanding non-cycling fibrous streamers (focal atrichia) vs. fibrotic tracts in scarring alopecia (Figure 11.13).

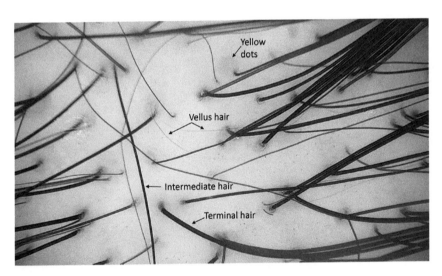

FIGURE 11.2 There is clear hair shaft variability in this case of AGA (×40).

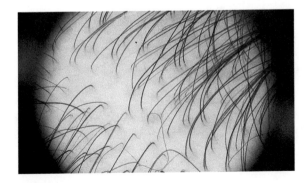

FIGURE 11.3 Most follicular units contain single hairs. Note the irregular pigmented network due to sun-induced hyperpigmentation of the scalp (×20).

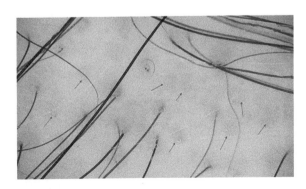

FIGURE 11.4 Yellow dots in frontal scalp in androgenetic alopecia (×40).

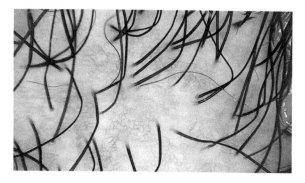

FIGURE 11.5 White peripilar sign in patient with AGA skin type IV.

PEARLS

- The biopsy should be obtained from the parietal scalp and not from the frontal scalp as this area is characterized by increased vellus/intermediate follicles, which can unmask the true terminal:vellus ratio.
- Trichoscopy should be used to select the optimal site for the biopsy to rule out focal LPP/FAPD.
- Diffuse alopecia in women can have more than one cause. Pathology can help to detect if there is follicular miniaturization and increased telogen count, which then has to be correlated with the clinical presentation.

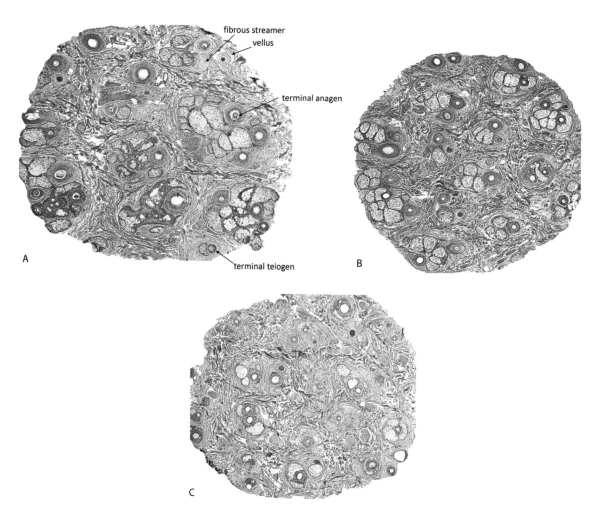

FIGURE 11.6 (A) In this biopsy, there are 11 follicular units, 8 terminal anagen, 1 telogen and 11 vellus follicles. The terminal:vellus ratio is 0.8:1 and the telogen count is 11%. (B, C) More examples of AGA characterized by clear-cut follicular miniaturization.

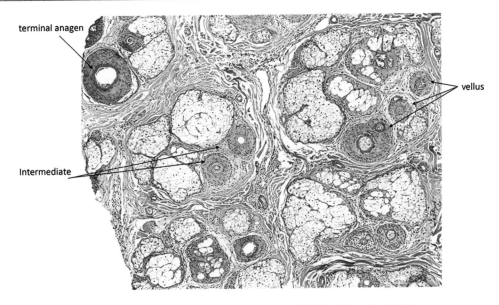

FIGURE 11.7 Androgenetic alopecia: the intermediate sized follicles are added to the vellus follicles.

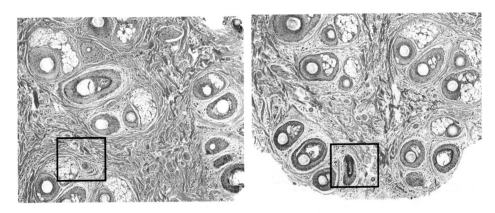

FIGURE 11.8 The black boxes demonstrate a small dermal papilla (A) that is visualized as a vellus follicle at further sections (B).

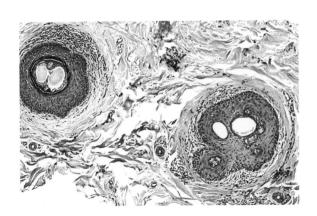

FIGURE 11.9 AGA: two compound follicles show perifollicular fibroplasia and lymphocytic infiltrate at the infundibulum. Note the preserved thickness of the follicular epithelium.

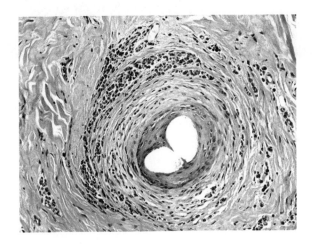

FIGURE 11.10 In lichen planopilaris, there is consumption (reduced thickness) of the follicular epithelium, layered perifollicular fibrosis and lichenoid inflammation. In this case, there is a pronounced plasma cell component.

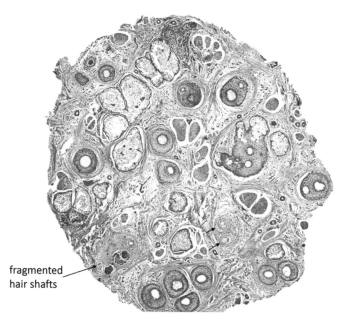

fragmented
hair shafts

FIGURE 11.11   Fragmented hair shafts (black arrows) in AGA.

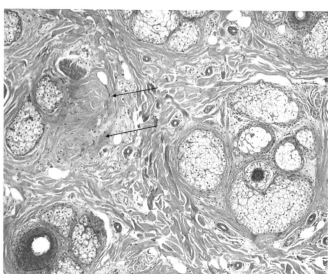

FIGURE 11.12   Advanced AGA with focal atrichia (arrows).

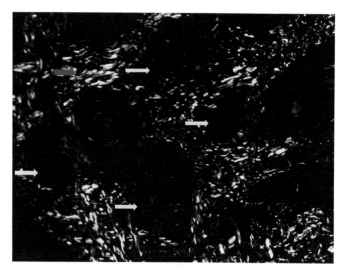

FIGURE 11.13   AGA with focal atrichia: the longstanding non-cycling fibrous streamers (yellow arrows) do not polarize compared to the true follicular scars in scarring alopecia, which polarize similarly to the interfollicular collagen of the dermis (red arrow).

FURTHER READING

Deloche C, de Lacharriere O, Misciali C, et al. Histological features of peripilar signs associated with androgenetic alopecia. Arch. Dermatol. Mar 2004;295(10):422–428.

Miteva M. A comprehensive approach to hair pathology of horizontal sections. J Am Acad Dermatol. Jul 2013;35(5):529–540.

Rudnicka, L, Oszewska M, Rakowska A, eds. *Atlas of Trichoscopy – Dermoscopy in Hair and Scalp Disease.* 1st ed. London: Springer-Verlag; 2012:221–222.

Whiting DA. Diagnostic and predictive value of horizontal sections of scalp biopsy specimens in male pattern androgenetic alopecia. J Am Acad Dermatol. May 1993;28(5 Pt 1):755–763.

Whiting DA. Scalp biopsy as a diagnostic and prognostic tool in androgenetic alopecia. Dermatol Ther. 1998;8(24):33.

Traumatic Alopecia (without Traction Alopecia)

12

Contents

TRICHOTILLOMANIA

GENERAL CONCEPTS

Trichotillomania (TM) is a form of traumatic alopecia characterized by round or bizarre areas of hair loss due to forceful pulling and plucking.

- A common clinical presentation of TM is decreased hair density (but rarely complete hair loss) on the crown in a tonsure pattern because this is an easily reachable area for the patient (Figure 12.1). The hairs are broken at different length and are surrounded by a rim of unaffected hair. Trichoteiromania (TR) (areas of hair loss due to rubbing of the scalp) presents in a similar way or as ill-defined patches of decreased hair density that can be associated with lichenification of the skin (see also Lichen Simplex Chronicus [LSC]).
- Repeated minor trauma to the follicles makes the hair shafts vulnerable to breakage in varying lengths.
- Main trichoscopic features include broken hairs of different length and various morphology resulting from the abrupt mechanical injury to anagen hairs (see also Chapter 1). These include flame hairs, tulip hairs, coiled hairs, exclamation mark hairs, hair powder sign, V-sign and burnt matchstick sign (Figures 12.2–12.4). Yellow dots can also be seen which correspond to empty follicular ostia containing only sebum and keratin. In TR, there can also be hair shafts displaying clean fractures (trichoptilosis), split ends (trichoclasis) and broom-like hairs (see also Figures 12.11–12.12) (Figure 12.5).

Main Histologic Features

In comparison to the histology of TR which is considered non-diagnostic, the histology of TM is well characterized and a scalp biopsy is helpful to exclude alopecia areata and to confirm the diagnosis. The forceful and strong plucking or pulling of hairs causes extraction of the hair shaft, trichomalacia, pigmented casts, detachment of the inner root sheath and empty hair canals.

- Normal or slightly decreased number of hair follicles with individual follicles or pairs of damaged follicles showing features of trichomalacia in 40% of the biopsies. *Trichomalacia* refers to hair shafts that are abnormal in shape and pigmentation, usually have a small diameter and/or are fragmented. Trichomalacia is not specific for TM, as it can be observed also in alopecia areata (Figures 12.6 and 12.7).

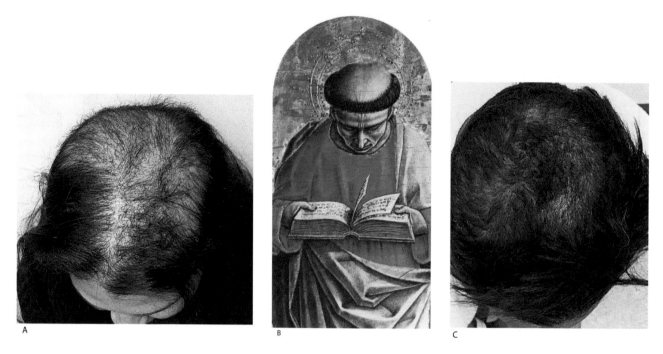

FIGURE 12.1 Tonsure pattern in trichotillomania (A) and trichoteiromania (C) is reminiscent of the monk's tonsure (B), where hair is shaved or cut on crown as a sign of religious devotion.

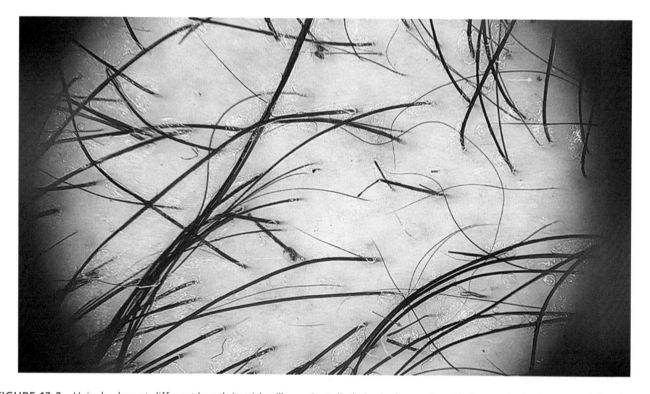

FIGURE 12.2 Hairs broken at different length in trichotillomania, tulip hairs (red arrow) and hair powder (yellow arrow) (×40).

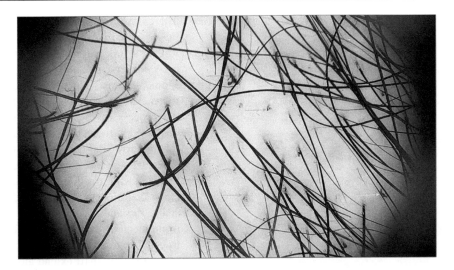

FIGURE 12.3   Hairs broken at different length in trichotillomania and flame hairs (red arrow), V-sign (blue arrow), coiled hairs (yellow arrow) and hair powder (green arrow).

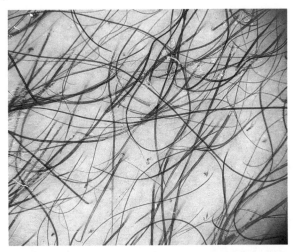

FIGURE 12.4   One-year-old girl with trichotillomania. Hairs are broken at different length and display different morphology (×40).

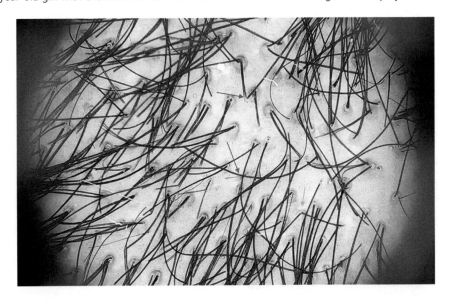

FIGURE 12.5   In trichoteiromania, hairs are broken at different length and they can show trichoptilosis (split ends) (red arrow), trichoclasis (clean hair shaft fracture with preserved cuticle) (green arrow) or broom-like fibers (blue arrow) as in lichen simplex chronicus.

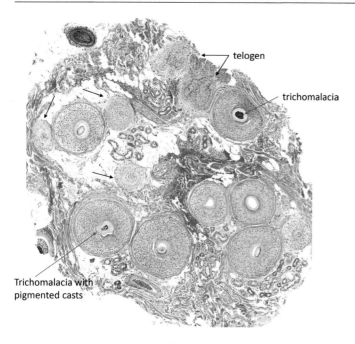

FIGURE 12.6 There are 31% follicles in catagen/telogen stage and two follicles show trichomalacia.

- There is catagen/telogen shift in up to 70% of the follicles (sometimes, the outer root sheath of an anagen follicle shows only a few apoptotic cells that mark early conversion to catagen (Figures 12.6 and 12.8).
- Pigmented casts – matrical or cortex cells containing melanin that are removed from the follicle by the process of forceful plucking. These cells are displaced in the upper hair canal where they shrink forming irregular black masses (Figures 12.6–12.8). They are not specific for TM and can be encountered in acute traction alopecia, central centrifugal cicatricial alopecia and dissecting cellulitis of the scalp. *Zip* and *button sign* are recognizable forms of pigmented casts. When the force is not as strong to cause extraction, the repeated minor pull forces make the hair shaft extend alone or with the inner root sheath. Initially, the pull forces disrupt the cortical substance with "reactive" linear aggregation of the melanin granules from the periphery in the center (when the vector of the force is upright) or at closer to the periphery (when the vector of the force is inclined) (Figure 12.9). This explains the *zip sign*.

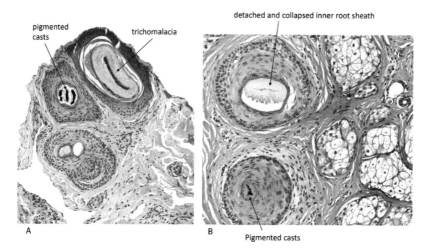

FIGURE 12.7 (A, B) Trichomalacia and pigmented casts.

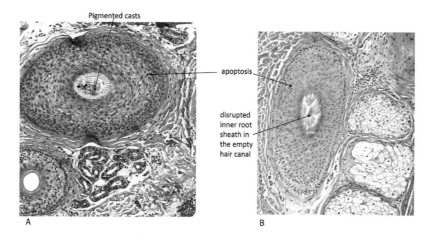

FIGURE 12.8 Traumatized anagen follicles undergoing catagen shift. Note the disrupted hair shaft morphology (A) and the empty hair canal (B).

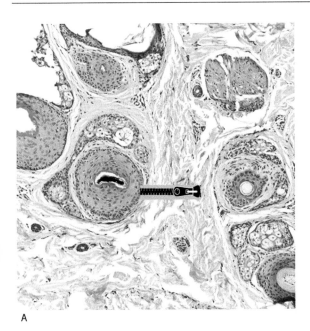
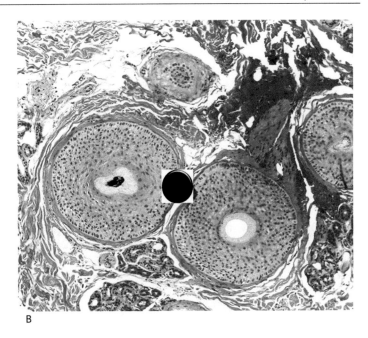

A

B

FIGURE 12.9   Pigmented casts: (A) the *zip* and (B) the *button sign*.

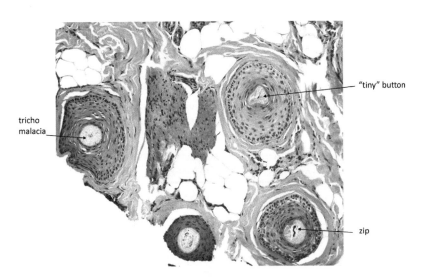

"tiny" button

tricho
malacia

zip

FIGURE 12.10   Another example of the *zip* and *button sign* in trichotillomania.

When the hair shaft extension reaches its tensile limit, the shaft either breaks off or/and is extracted from the follicle leaving just an aggregate of melanin granules surrounded by the collapsed inner root sheath (*button sign*) (Figures 12.9 and 12.10).

- Perifollicular hemorrhage near the follicular bulb or between the follicular sheaths.
- *Hamburger sign*: longitudinal breakage of the hair shaft with accumulation of proteinaceous material and red blood cells in the resulting cavity. This corresponds to hair shafts with split ends on trichoscopy (see Figure 12.16).

LICHEN SIMPLEX CHRONICUS

GENERAL CONCEPTS

- LSC is a chronic pruritic condition characterized by lichenified erythematous scaly plaques that occur as a result of constant scratching or rubbing of the skin and the scalp is one of the most common locations.
- Repeated trauma to the follicles from rubbing and scratching makes the hair shafts vulnerable to breakage in varying lengths as well as to splitting at their ends.

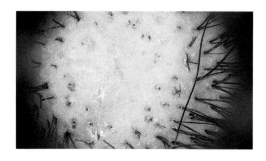

FIGURE 12.11   Dry trichoscopy shows white scale, focal hemorrhagic crust and broom-like hairs (×60).

- On trichoscopy, there are short hair shafts emerging as a single stem from a follicular opening, which show proximal split into two or three hairs of similar

thickness at the level of the surface and hair shafts of same characteristics but with additional distal split of the hair tips into two or three tiny hair endings (*broom hairs*) (Figures 12.11 and 12.12). There are dotted vessels arranged in swirling lines (string of pearls) similar to clear cell acanthoma (Figure 12.12).

Main Histologic Features

- Epidermal hyperplasia with irregular lengthening of the rete ridges, orthokeratosis and hypergranulosus on vertical sections (Figure 12.13).
- Overall preserved follicular architecture, normal number of terminal follicles but with increased

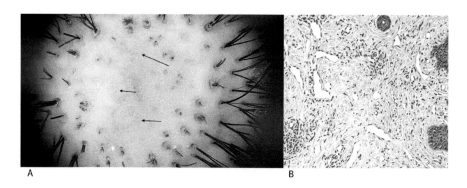

A   B

FIGURE 12.12   Using an alcohol gel helps to hydrate the scale and visualize the dotted vessels arranged in linear strings (A, black arrow) (×60) that correspond to increased number of dilated capillaries on pathology (B).

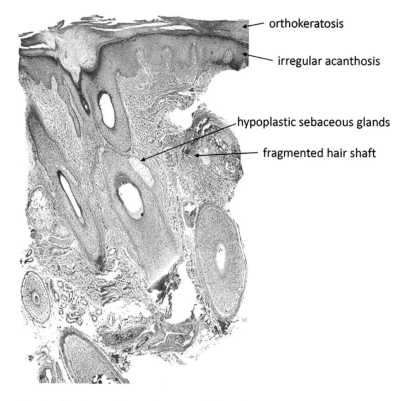

orthokeratosis

irregular acanthosis

hypoplastic sebaceous glands

fragmented hair shaft

FIGURE 12.13   Lichen simplex chronicus of the scalp on vertical sections.

catagen/telogen count and diminished in size and number sebaceous glands.

- The *gear wheel* sign representing the jagged acanthotic projections of the outer root sheaths around the hair canal at the level of the infundibulum on horizontal sections (Figure 12.14).
- Infundibular hyperkeratosis (Figure 12.15).
- *Hamburger sign*: longitudinal breakage of the hair shaft with accumulation of proteinaceous material and red blood cells in the resulting cavity (Figure 12.16).
- Fragmented (naked) hairs shafts with granulomatous inflammation can be found in the dermis (Figure 12.13).

PRESSURE-INDUCED AND POSTOPERATIVE ALOPECIA

GENERAL CONCEPTS

- Postoperative alopecia results from extensive external pressure leading to ischemic changes in the hair follicles, usually in patients that undergo lengthy operations or who are immobilized. It generally manifests as a circumscribed alopecic area in the

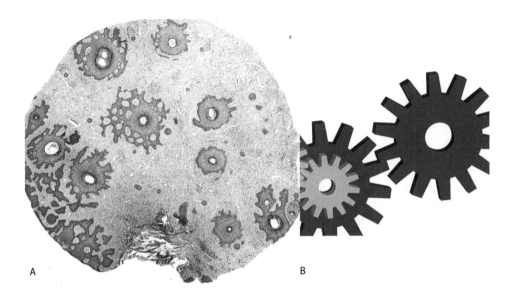

A   B

FIGURE 12.14   Jagged acanthotic projections of the outer root sheaths resemble (B) gear wheels in LSC.

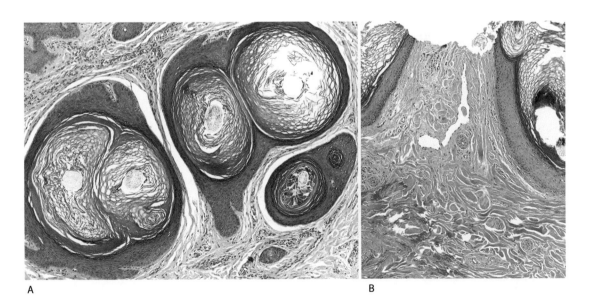

A   B

FIGURE 12.15   (A) Dilated ostia with infundibular hyperkeratosis and dilated bizarre-shaped vessels with prominent, plump endothelial cells (B).

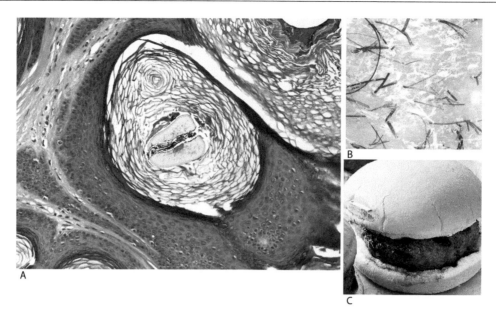

FIGURE 12.16 (A) In LSC, the hamburger sign (C) corresponds to split hair shafts. The hair shaft is split in two, as shown on the trichoscopic image (B) and contains proteinaceous material and red blood cells.

occipital scalp and can be preceded by tenderness or swelling (Figure 12.17).

- Both scarring and non-scarring alopecia have been reported. Pressure-induced alopecia can progress to permanent alopecia and the most significant factor in prognosis might be the duration of the operation time.
- Occipital pressure-induced alopecia has also been reported as pressure ulcers in military personnel admitted to a polytrauma rehabilitation center. We have observed a pressure-induced alopecia after

tightly placed stitches in a scalp biopsy, which got secondary staphylococcal infection. (Figure 12.18).

- On trichoscopy, there are broken hairs at different levels, black dots and yellow dots (Figure 12.17).

Main Histologic Features

- An increased number of catagen/telogen follicles (Figure 12.19).
- An increased number of anagen follicles with apoptotic cells (catagen shift) due to hypoxia.

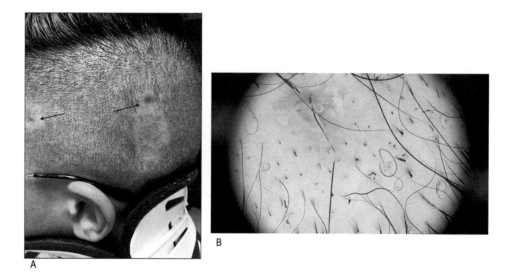

FIGURE 12.17 (A) Pressure-induced alopecia on both sides due to the prolonged attachment of a halo brace after surgery. (B) On trichoscopy, there are broken hairs at different lengths, flame hairs, hair powder and yellow dots.

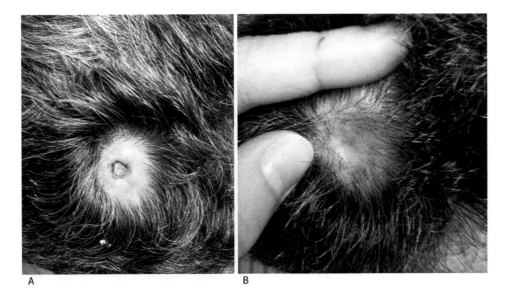

FIGURE 12.18   (A) A newly developed patch of pressure-induced alopecia due to tight sutures after biopsy and secondary infection. (B) Some regrowth is noted after 6 weeks.

- Trichomalacia and syringometaplasia (Figure 12.20). Syringometaplasia is an adaptive, benign process of the eccrine ducts and glands in response to the trauma and hypoxia.
- The epidermis can be normal, hyperplastic or ulcerated. Chronic inflammation and foreign body granulomatous infiltrate can be observed too (see Figure 12.19).

PEARLS

- Pigmented casts within the hair canals of vellus follicles favor alopecia areata over trichotillomania
- Trichotillomania may be indistinguishable from acute traction alopecia on histology.

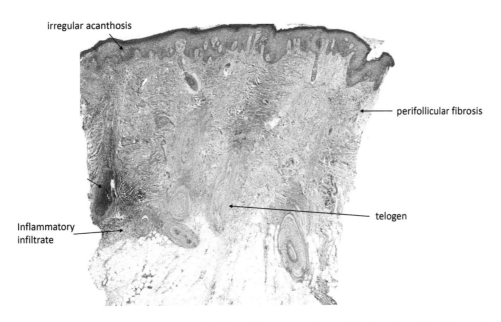

FIGURE 12.19   This case of pressure-induced alopecia developed due to wearing a tight bandage following scalp surgery. Note the increased telogen count, inflammation and acanthosis as reactive phenomena to the trauma.

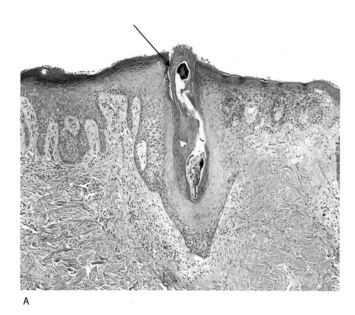

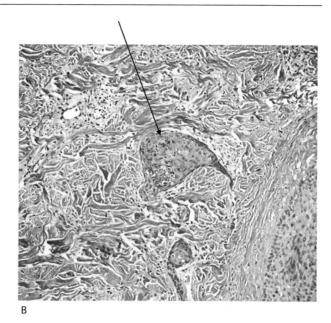

A   B

FIGURE 12.20   Further sections of the same case (Figure 12.19) showing (A) trichomalacia and (B) squamous syringometaplasia (arrows) due to prolonged hypoxia.

FURTHER READING

Bergfeld W, Mulinari-Brenner F, McCarron K, Embi C. The combined utilization of clinical and histological findings in the diagnosis of trichotillomania. J Cutan Pathol. Apr 2002;29(4):207–14.

Davies KE, Yesudian P. Pressure alopecia. Int J Trichology. 2012 Apr;4(2):64–8.

Freyschmidt-Paul P, Hoffmann R, Happle R. Trichoteiromania. Eur J Dermatol. Jul–Aug 2001;11(4):369–71.

Hanly AJ, Jorda M, Badiavas E, Valencia I, Elgart GW. Postoperative pressure-induced alopecia: report of a case and discussion of the role of apoptosis in non-scarring alopecia. J Cutan Pathol. Aug 1999;26(7):357–61.

Loh SH, Lew BL, Sim WY. Pressure alopecia: clinical findings and prognosis. J Am Acad Dermatol. 2015 Jan;72(1):188–9. Dermoscopy Made Simple: http://dermoscopymadesimple. blogspot.com/

Miteva M, Romanelli P, Tosti A. Pigmented casts. Am J Dermatopathol. 2014 Jan;36(1):58–63.

Muller SA. Trichotillomania: a histopathologic study in sixty-six patients. J Am Acad Dermatol. 1990 Jul;23(1):56–62.

Quaresma MV, Mariño Alvarez AM, Miteva M. Dermatoscopic-pathologic correlation of lichen simplex chronicus on the scalp: 'broom fibres, gear wheels and hamburgers'. J Eur Acad Dermatol Venereol. 2016;30:343–5.

Rakowska A, Slowinska M, Olszewska M, Rudnicka L. New trichoscopy findings in trichotillomania: flame hairs, V-sign, hook hairs, hair powder, tulip hairs. Acta Derm Venereol. 2014 May;94(3):303–6.

Royer MC, Sperling LC. Splitting hairs: the 'hamburger sign' in trichotillomania. J Cutan Pathol. Sep 2006;33 Suppl 2:63–4.

Lichen Planopilaris

13

Contents

GENERAL CONCEPTS

Lichen planopilaris (LPP), a follicular form of lichen planus (LP), is a primary lymphocytic cicatricial alopecia characterized by irreversible hair loss and scarring.

- Several mechanisms have been implicated involving deficient peroxisome proliferator-activated receptor (PPAR) followed by destruction of the pilosebaceous unit, CD-8$^+$ T-cell-induced apoptosis of the epithelial follicular stem cells (eHFSCs) that have lost their immune privilege (IP) and epithelial mesenchymal transition of the follicular eHFSCs, which have survived the massive apoptosis. The bulge IP collapse in LPP shows striking similarity to the bulb IP collapse in alopecia areata.

- Clinically, several subtypes have been described including *patchy* (one or more patches that start on vertex and expand (Figure 13.1), *diffuse* (the vertex is initially affected but patches can occur anywhere), *patterned* or *fibrosing alopecia in a pattern distribution* (FAPD) (overlap between diffuse LPP and androgenetic alopecia). Other forms include *linear LPP* (Figure 13.1), which can simulate morphea *en coup du sabre* and linear lupus profundus; *Graham-Little-Picardi-Lasseur* syndrome (a triad of LPP on scalp, non-scarring alopecia of the axillary and

pubic hair, and widespread follicular papules – lichen planus spinulosus); LPP can also rarely occur in children where it is usually misdiagnosed as alopecia areata or tinea capitis on clinical exam (Figure 13.2). The main differential diagnosis includes keratosis follicularis spinulosa decalvans (KFSD), which is a rare genetic condition of X-linked inheritance (but sporadic and autosomal dominant cases may occur), with onset during childhood that presents with keratotic follicular papules on the body, scarring alopecia on the scalp, eyebrows and progresses over puberty (Figure 13.3). *Hypopigmented macules on scalp with associated alopecia* have been reported as a subtype of LPP on the scalp in African American patients (Figure 13.4).

- LPP can be associated with frontal fibrosing alopecia (FFA) in 16–21% of the cases. FFA and FAPD are discussed in Chapters 14 and 15.

- Folliculitis decalvans lichen planopilaris phenotypic spectrum (FDLPPPS) refers to cases of lymphocytic scarring alopecia showing dual clinical, trichoscopic and histologic features for FD and LPP (see below).

- LPP can be underdiagnosed prior to hair transplant if not biopsied and this could lead to loss of the follicular grafts after hair transplant (see Figure 13.17).

- On *trichoscopy,* there are loss of follicular openings, peripilar casts (tubular scales entangling the proximal 2–3 mm of the hair shaft emergences

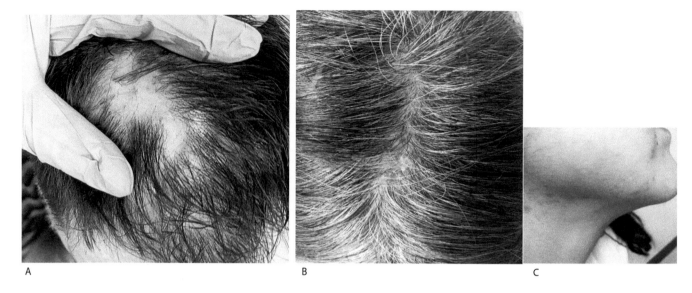

FIGURE 13.1 (A) Patchy LPP and (B, C) linear LPP on the scalp and face in another patient.

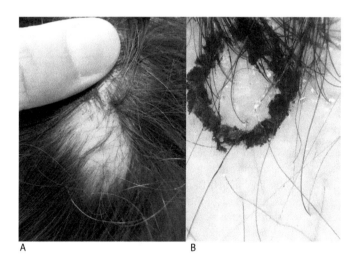

FIGURE 13.2 (A) A case of biopsy proven LPP in a 10-year-old child that has been misdiagnosed as tinea capitis. (B) The site of trichoscopy-guided scalp biopsy shows peripilar casts (×10).

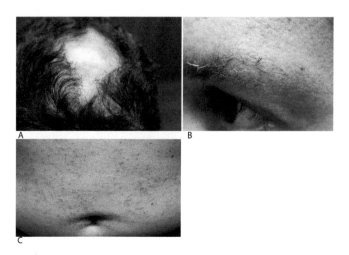

FIGURE 13.3 (A–C) Keratosis follicularis spinulosa decalvans.

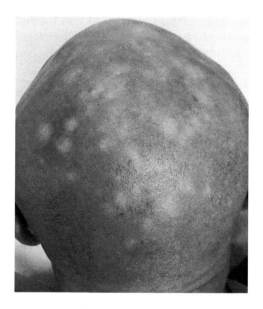

FIGURE 13.4 Hypopigmented LPP in an African American patient.

(Figure 13.5), elongated linear blood vessels (Figure 13.6), tufts of hairs (usually 2–4 hairs emerging from the same ostium and surrounded by peripilar casts) (Figure 13.6). In skin types IV-VI, there are blue-gray dots in a target pattern that correspond to pigment incontinence in follicular proximity vs. blue-gray dots in a speckled pattern in discoid lupus erythematosus (DLE) that correspond to interfollicular interface pattern with pigment incontinence (Figure 13.7). White dots correspond to fibrotic tracts replacing individual follicular ostia usually at the margin of the active patch (Figure 13.8) and milky white areas (strawberry ice cream color) correspond to larger areas of follicular scarring.

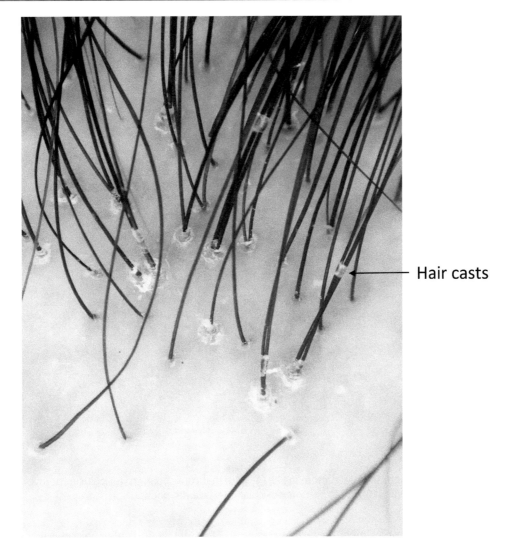

Hair casts

FIGURE 13.5 Peripilar tubular casts encircling the proximal portions of the hair shafts. Hair casts (arrow) are noted along the length of some hair shafts (×10).

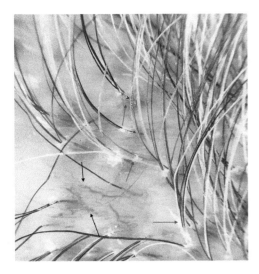

FIGURE 13.6 Linear vessels in LPP (black arrow) and tufts of 2–3 hairs coming out of the same emergence (red arrow) (×10).

MAIN HISTOLOGIC FEATURES

- Decreased number of follicles, altered follicular architecture with areas of follicular dropout and absent/diminished number of sebaceous glands (Figure 13.9). Sebaceous gland inflammation, including sebaceous duct inflammation, is usually an early feature of primary scarring alopecia (Figure 13.10).
- "Eyes and goggles" can be recognized on low power. These are compound follicular structures assessed at the level of the isthmus or below (see Chapter 6) (Figure 13.11).
- Perifollicular lichenoid/interface lymphocytic infiltrate involving the permanent portion of the hair follicle (isthmus and infundibulum). The infiltrate can show also interface pattern (invading the outer root sheath) (Figures 13.12 and 13.13).

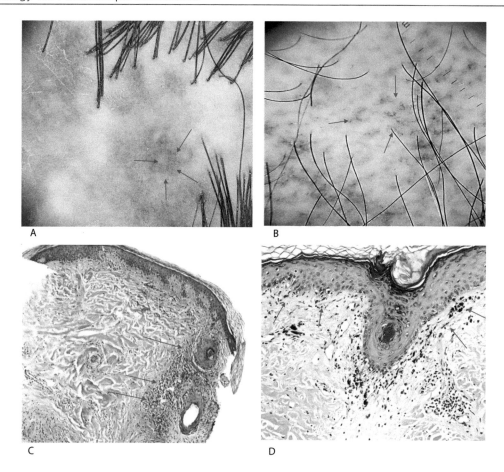

FIGURE 13.7   Blue-gray dots in a peripilar target pattern in LPP (A, ×40) that corresponds to folliculocentric involvement on histology (C), and in a speckled pattern in DLE (B, ×10) due to the interfollicular interface dermatitis (D).

- Perifollicular concentric fibrosis (onion-like layered fibrosis) involving the permanent portion of the hair follicle. There may be increased mucin (mucinous fibrosis) (Figure 13.12).
- There is consumption of the follicular epithelium (thinning of the outer root sheath) (Figure 13.12)

vs. intact follicular epithelium in cases of AGA with follicular inflammation and fibroplasia (see Chapter 11).
- Follicular scars (dropout) with fragmented hair shafts (Figure 13.12).

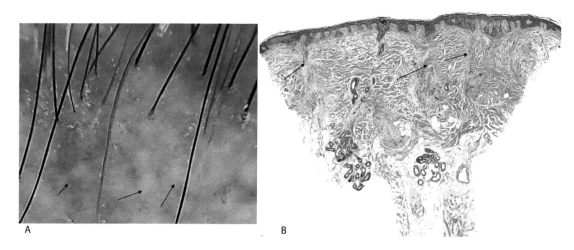

FIGURE 13.8   (A) White dots on trichoscopy (×10) corresponding to (B) the fibrotic tracts replacing the existing follicles on histology (arrows).

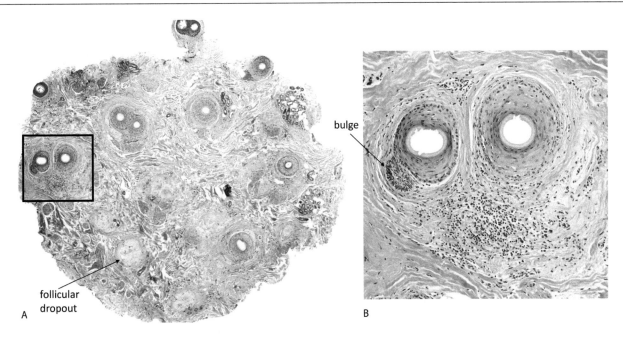

FIGURE 13.9 (A) Altered follicular architecture with areas of follicular dropout, absent sebaceous glands and lichenoid infiltrate at the permanent portion of the hair follicle (the bulge), as shown in (B).

FOLLICULITIS DECALVANS LICHEN PLANOPILARIS PHENOTYPIC SPECTRUM (FDLPPPS)

These are cases of patchy or diffuse lymphocytic scarring alopecia that present with ambiguous features for FD and LPP, which makes stratifying the diagnosis difficult.

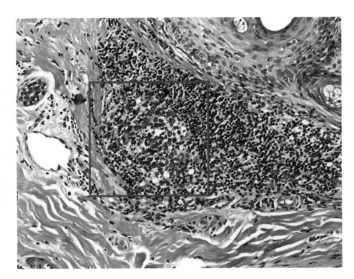

FIGURE 13.10 Lichenoid inflammatory infiltrate involving the sebaceous lobules.

- Main features:
  - Polytrichia (Figure 13.14)
  - Positive bacterial culture for *Staphylococcus* from pustules and hemorrhagic crusts
  - "Mixed" histologic features for primary cicatricial alopecia including multicompound follicular structures of average 2–5 follicles (follicular packs), atrophy of the follicular epithelium, lymphohistiocytic infiltrate with granulomas and prominent plasma cells, but absence of neutrophilic infiltrate (Figures 13.15 and 13.16)
  - Clinical improvement with systemic antimicrobials and immunomodulatory agents
- *Caveat:* FD in chronic stage or in remission can present with polytrichia and lack of neutrophils but plasma cells on histology, therefore some consider FDLPPPS as a continuum of FD with concomitant lichenoid features.

UNDERRECOGNIZING LPP IN THE PATTERNED AREA IS A PITFALL FOR HAIR TRANSPLANT IN ANDROGENETIC ALOPECIA (AGA)

- Early/subtle LPP may co-exist with AGA but maybe underdiagnosed if patients are asymptomatic, and trichoscopy and histology are not utilized to

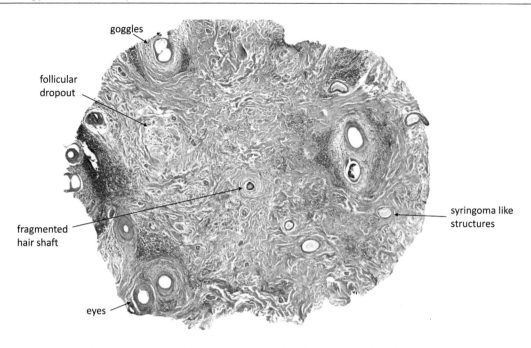

goggles

follicular
dropout

fragmented
hair shaft

syringoma like
structures

eyes

FIGURE 13.11   Eyes and goggles (compound follicles) with perifollicular fibrosis and lichenoid infiltrate.

exclude the diagnosis. This pitfall is more common in patients presenting with FAPD.

- Using trichosopy to detect individual hairs or tufts of hairs with peripilar casts is critical to suspect the diagnosis of subtle LPP and to guide the optimal site for the biopsy (Figure 13.17).

- Failure to diagnose subtle LPP in patients undergoing hair transplant for AGA can result in catastrophic loss of follicular grafts.

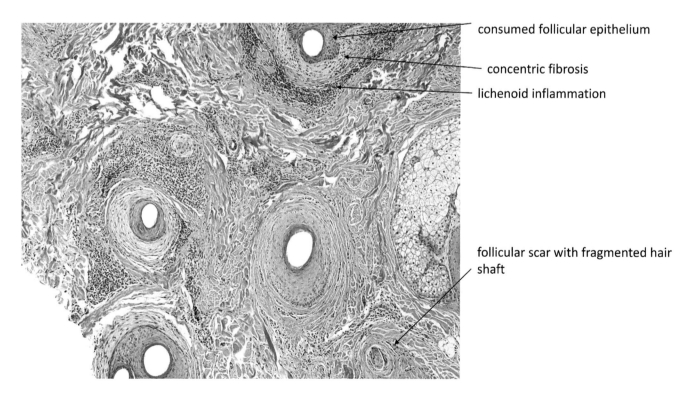

consumed follicular epithelium

concentric fibrosis

lichenoid inflammation

follicular scar with fragmented hair shaft

FIGURE 13.12   Perifollicular fibrosis and lichenoid inflammation at the upper follicular level. Note the consumption (thinning) of the outer root sheath in the involved follicles.

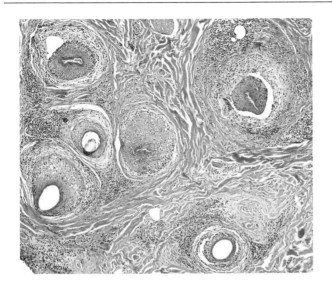

FIGURE 13.13 Interface (invading within the follicular epithelium) lymphocytic infiltrate in LPP.

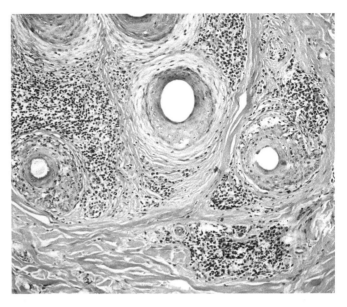

FIGURE 13.16 Plasma cell infiltrate in FDLPPPS.

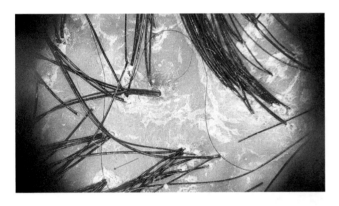

FIGURE 13.14 Polytrichia (big tufts) with peripilar casts, interfollicular scaling and a yellow crust (×40) in a patient FDLPPPS (the bacterial culture was positive for *S. aureus*).

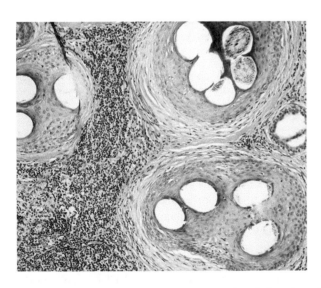

FIGURE 13.15 Polytrichia (multi-compound follicles) with perifollicular fibrosis and lichenoid infiltrate of lymphocytes, histiocytes and plasma cells. Note the absence of neutrophils.

OVERDIAGNOSING LPP IN BIOPSIES FROM THE RECIPIENT AREA OF PATIENTS WITH FOLLICULAR GRAFT LOSS IS A HISTOLOGIC PITFALL

- This is not uncommon in my experience. If the hair transplant surgeon/trichologist submits a scalp biopsy from the recipient area with graft loss with the rule out diagnosis LPP, the histologic diagnosis is usually "confirmed". This may result in unnecessary treatments, psychologic aggravation, financial loss and delay in the repeat hair transplant procedure.
- There are usually no peripilar casts but area of focal atrichia may be detected (Figure 13.18).
- Several biopsies for horizontal sections should be obtained following the guidelines for trichoscopy-guided biopsies (as for LPP) to increase the diagnostic yield.
- On histology, there may be follicular dropout (corresponding to loss of follicular grafts), fragmented hairs shafts with granulomatous infiltrate but otherwise overall preserved follicular architecture with intact sebaceous glands, no perifollicular fibrosis and lichenoid infiltrate (Figure 13.19). The follicles appear less grouped in follicular units.

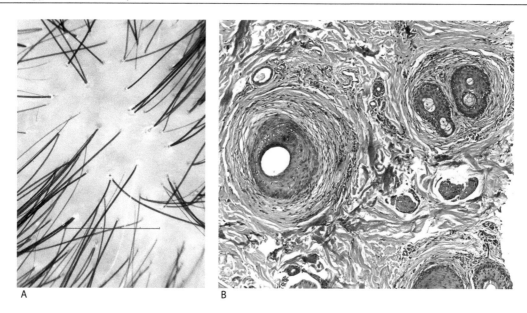

FIGURE 13.17 LPP in a patient with AGA suspected on trichoscopy (A, ×10) by the presence of peripilar casts and small tufts of hairs and confirmed on histology (B).

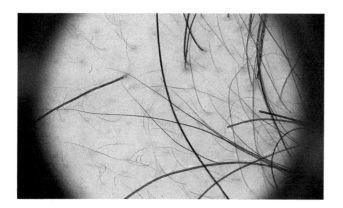

FIGURE 13.18 This patient with hair loss after hair transplant was overdiagnosed with LPP/FFA in the temporal scalp.

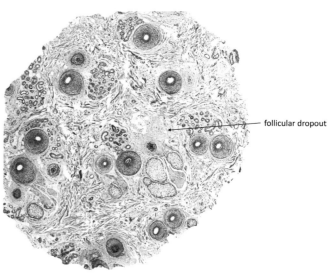

follicular dropout

FIGURE 13.19 AGA misdiagnosed as LPP after hair transplant in a patient with follicular graft loss.

PEARLS

- Trichoscopy-guided biopsies sectioned as horizontal sections have a higher diagnostic yield in scarring alopecia, including LPP, and should be obtained from the tufts, or the hairs with peripilar casts and peripilar blue-gray dots. They allow for appreciation of the follicular architecture and for spotting subtle/focal disease.
- Perieccrine lymphocytic infiltrate is not specific for discoid lupus erythematosus and can occasionally be seen in other cicatricial alopecias including LPP (Figure 13.20).
- The lymphocytic infiltrate involving the lower portion of the hair follicle in the fat can be misinterpreted as the swarm of bees infiltrate in alopecia areata.

- LPP can be indistinguishable from FFA on H&E sections. Some histologic features that favor FFA include pronounced apoptosis in the outer root sheath, the inflammation and fibrosis extend below the isthmus, and the inflammatory infiltrate affects simultaneously anagen, telogen and vellus follicles. A recent work found statistically significant greater numbers of CD68+ cells in the peri-follicular mesenchyme at the bulge and infundibulum in LPP vs. FFA.

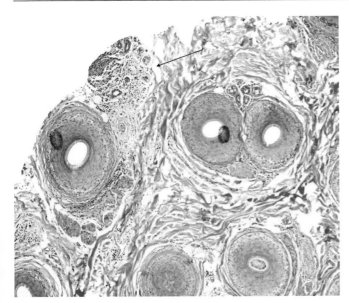

FIGURE 13.20 Perieccrine lymphocytic infiltrate in a biopsy from LPP.

FURTHER READING

Al-Zaid T, Vanderweil S, Zembowicz A, Lyle S. Sebaceous gland loss and inflammation in scarring alopecia: a potential role in pathogenesis. J Am Acad Dermatol. 2011 Sep;65(3):597–603.

Baquerizo Nole KL, Nusbaum B, Pinto GM, Miteva M. Lichen planopilaris in the androgenetic alopecia area: a pitfall for hair transplantation. Skin Appendage Disord. 2015 Mar;1(1):49–53.

Desai N, Mirmirani P. Lichen planopilaris. In Miteva M, ed. *Alopecia*. 1st ed. Elsevier, 2018: 143–150.

Harries M, Hardman J, Chaudhry I, Poblet E, Paus R. Profiling the human hair follicle immune system in lichen planopilaris and frontal fibrosing alopecia: can macrophage polarization differentiate these two conditions microscopically? Br J Dermatol. 2019 Dec 28. doi: 10.1111/bjd.18854.

Harries, MJ, Meyer K, Chaudhry I, Poblet EKJE, Griffiths CE, Paus R. Lichen planopilaris is characterized by immune privilege collapse of the hair follicle's epithelial stem cell niche. J Pathol. 2013;231(2):236–247.

Imanishi, H, Ansell DM, Cheret J, Harries M, Bertolini M, Sepp N, Biro T, Poblet E, Jimenez F, Hardman J, Panicker SP, Ward CM, Paus R. Epithelial-to-mesenchymal stem cell transition in a human organ: lessons from lichen planopilaris. J Invest Dermatol. 2018;138(3):511–519.

Karnik P, Tekeste Z, McCormick TS, Gilliam AC, Price VH, Cooper KD, Mirmirani P. Hair follicle stem cell-specific PPARgamma deletion causes scarring alopecia. J Invest Dermatol. 2009; 129(5):1243–1257.

Miteva M, Tosti A. Dermoscopy guided scalp biopsy in cicatricial alopecia. J Eur Acad Dermatol Venereol. 2013;27(10):1299–1303.

Olszewska M, Rakowska A, Slowinska M, Rudnicka L. Classic lichen planopilaris and Graham Little syndrome. In Rudnicka L, Olszewksa M, Rakowska A, ed. *Atlas of Trichoscopy*. 1st ed. Springer-Verlag, London, 2012: 279–294.

Frontal Fibrosing Alopecia

14

Contents

GENERAL CONCEPTS

Frontal Fibrosing Alopecia (FFA) is a progressive lymphocytic scarring alopecia characterized by a band-like area of frontal or frontotemporal hairline recession most commonly in post-menopausal women. Eyebrows, eyelashes, and sideburns as well as limb, axillary, moustache, beard, and pubic hair involvement can be present too. The dermatological literature is currently exploding in papers on FFA, therefore this chapter aims to summarize curious/novel trichoscopic-pathologic correlations.

- The pathogenesis of FFA is unclear but considered to be overlapping with lichen planopilaris (LPP) (see Lichen Planopilaris). Recent genome-wide association study showed that FFA is a genetically predisposed immuno-inflammatory disorder driven by HLA-B*07:02 allele on chromosome 6.
- There are three *most common* clinical patterns: (1) a linear uniform band of hair loss of the frontal hairline, (2) an irregular or zigzag pattern at and behind the frontal hairline, and (3) a 'pseudo-fringe-sign pattern' with hair loss behind the preserved frontal hairline. Several *unusual variants* have been identified including: (1) androgenetic alopecia-like pattern, (2) cockade-like pattern, and (3) ophiasis-like pattern (Figure 14.1). Other unusual variants include occipital FFA, patchy FFA and upsilon-like FFA.
- Two curious associations: *Lichen planus pigmentosus (LPPigm)* is more prevalent in FFA patients with darker skin, can precede the diagnosis and presents as brown macules coalescing into patches on the face and upper trunk; *(yellow) facial papules* are skin-colored monotonous papules on the face, usually the temporal and malar area. Both features have been found more prevalent among premenopausal and Hispanic/Latino women (Figure 14.2).
- On *trichoscopy* the features are similar to LPP (see Chapter 13). Some additional or distinct features include:
  - Loss of vellus hairs in the hairline (Figure 14.3A): while this is the rule, there can be exceptional/early cases of retained vellus hairs (Figure 14.3B)
  - Lack of tufts (compound hairs) compared to LPP (unpublished data; personal communication with Dr. Giselle Martins); the histologic correlation to this is that in FFA there are usually "eyes" and not "goggles" (see Figure 14.10)
  - Peripilar casts are usually more subtle and absent in the sideburns (Figure 14.4)
  - Vessel net (this corresponds to the superficial vascular plexus with its branching vessels visualized by trichoscopy due to the atrophy of the skin) (Figure 14.5)
  - Peripilar hypopigmented halo (Figure 14.6)
  - Eyebrow trichoscopy can show yellow dots, dystrophic hairs, gray dots and hairs growing in different directions (Figure 14.7). Trichochorrhexis nodosa can also be observed most likely due to aggressive topical application (personal observation) (Figure 14.8)
  - LPPigm: folliculocentric blue-gray dots in circles, speckled dots, and rhomboid structures (Figure 14.9). In melasma the pigment is not folliculocentric

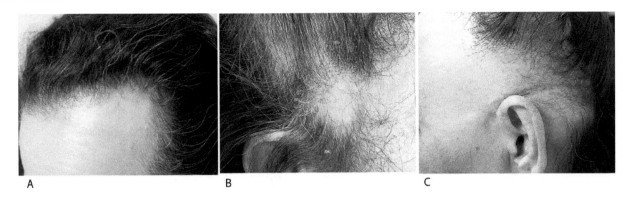

FIGURE 14.1   The 3 unusual clinical subtypes in FFA: (A) AGA-like pattern, (B) cockade, and (C) ophiasis pattern.

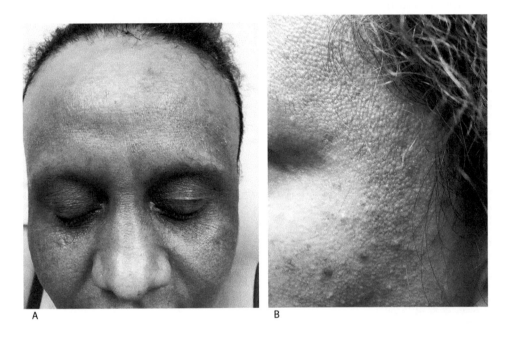

FIGURE 14.2   Two curious associations with FFA: (A) LPPigm (diffuse brown patches on face, note involvement of the upper eyelids) and (B) yellow facial papules.

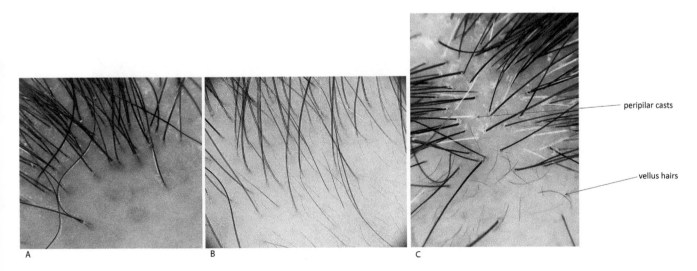

FIGURE 14.3   Loss of vellus hairs in the frontal line in FFA (A) compared to normal hairline (B, ×20). (C) FFA with preserved vellus hairs but peripilar casts in the immediate vicinity behind (×10).

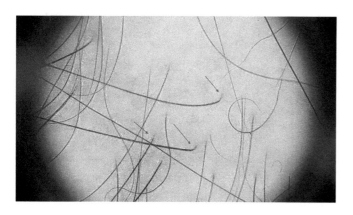

FIGURE 14.4 Preauricular areas/sideburns show lack of peripilar casts but transparent proximal emergences (×20).

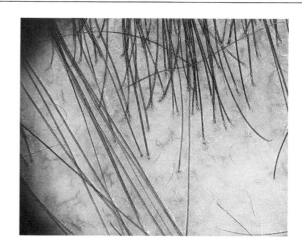

FIGURE 14.5 Vessel net in FFA (×40).

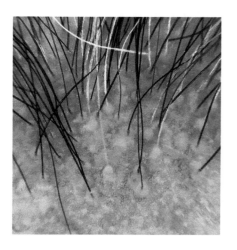

FIGURE 14.6 Peripilar hypopigmented halo in FFA (×10).

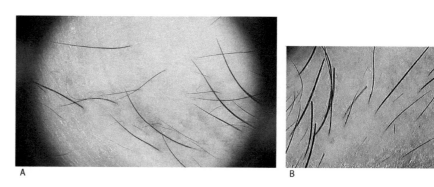

FIGURE 14.7 (A) Eyebrow trichoscopy in FFA: yellow, gray dots and hair growing in distinct directions. (B) Dystrophic hairs: this patient has not plucked the eyebrows within last 6 months (×40).

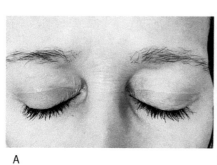

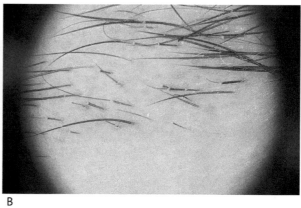

FIGURE 14.8 (A) Trichorrhexis nodosa of the eyebrows in FFA. The patient has been rubbing pimecrolimus cream into the affected eyebrows (B, ×20).

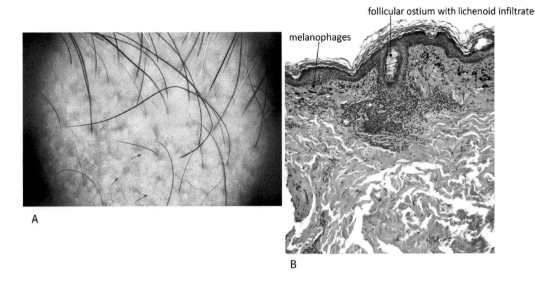

FIGURE 14.9   (A) LPPigm on the forehead extending to the frontal hairline in FFA shows blue-gray dots in circles (×50) which is a clue to (B) periappendigeal involvement with accentuation of melanophages.

MAIN HISTOLOGIC FEATURES

- The histologic features may be *indistinguishable* from LPP on H&E sections (see Chapter 13). Histologic features, more pertinent to FFA include:
  - There is usually more pronounced follicular apoptosis and clefting between the follicular epithelium and the zone of fibrosis compared to LPP (Figure 14.10)
  - The follicular triad is a clue to the diagnosis of FFA: it refers to the simultaneous involvement of terminal anagen, telogen and vellus follicles (Figure 14.11)

- *Early cases of FFA* show the "inflammatory pattern": in early FFA there is a lack of perifollicular fibrosis and lichenoid inflammation of the terminal follicles. The inflammatory involvement of the vellus follicles by perifollicular lichenoid layered or patchy infiltrate and the atrophy of the sebaceous glands is the histologic clue to the diagnosis. There is usually hypoplasia of the sebaceous glands (Figure 14.12).
- Biopsies from FFA involving the *limbs* show similar inflammatory pattern with lack of perifollicular fibrosis. In longstanding cases, in which the follicles are missing, solitary arrector pili muscle bundles are noted in the dermis (Figure 14.13B).

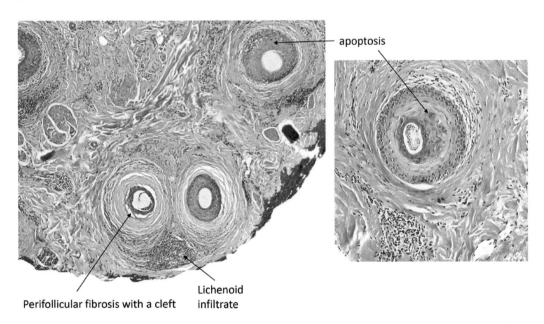

FIGURE 14.10   FFA demonstrating the more pronounced clefting and apoptosis.

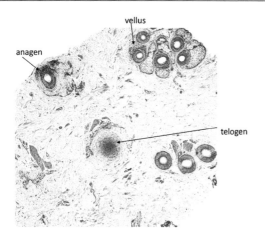

FIGURE 14.11 The follicular triad is the simultaneous involvement of vellus, terminal anagen and telogen follicles.

- *Eyebrows:* In the eyebrows the hair follicles are single and are not organized in follicular units. Most of the follicles are in telogen phase. Several patterns can be observed in the biopsies: (1) inflammatory pattern that needs to be distinguished from alopecia areata by the level of the lymphocytic inflammation (the isthmus and infundibulum in FFA vs. the bulb in alopecia areata), (2) perifollicular fibrosis with lichenoid inflammation (Figure 14.14A,B) and (3) follicular scarring (fibrotic tracts) that extend up to the surface and correlate with the white areas on trichoscopy (Figure 14.14D). This feature also explains the regrowth of hairs in distinct directions as the existing follicles need to reorient their growth in a new direction to avoid the fibrotic tracts.

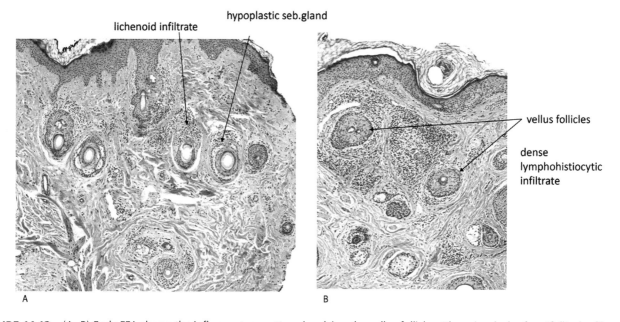

FIGURE 14.12 (A, B) Early FFA shows the inflammatory pattern involving the vellus follicles. There is a lack of perifollicular fibrosis.

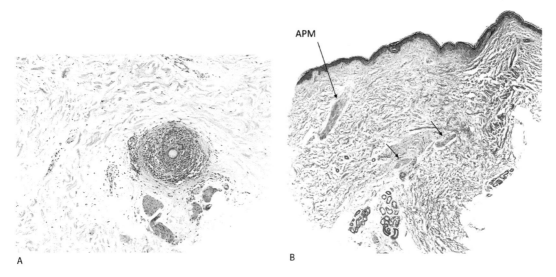

FIGURE 14.13 (A) Inflammatory infiltrate involving a telogen follicle in the dermis in a biopsy from patchy alopecia of the forearm in a man with FFA. (B) Another example from FFA of the forearm: no follicles are present, only solitary arrector pili muscle (APM) bundles in the dermis.

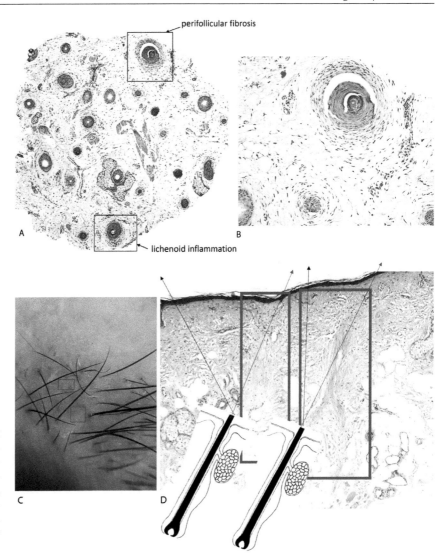

perifollicular fibrosis

lichenoid inflammation

A

B

C

D

FIGURE 14.14 (A, B) Eyebrow involvement in FFA reveals individual follicles with perifollicular fibrosis and lichenoid inflammation. Note that the follicles are not organized in follicular units. (C, D) Eyebrow involvement in FFA reveals fibrotic tracts extending to the surface (replacing the viable follicles). The interposition of this scar tissue may be the reason why the hairs grow in distinct directions.

- *LPPigm* may show follicular pattern in biopsies from FFA (see Figure 14.9). This involvement of the vellus follicles is curious as it may explain the association between FFA and LPPigm. The differential diagnosis of LPPigm includes pigmented contact dermatitis to Paraphenylenediamine (PPD), essential oils or fragrance (Figure 14.15).
- *Fibrous papules*: Based on the collected data from small number of biopsies two hypotheses are currently favored: (1) this is a lichenoid folliculitis involving the vellus follicles (16 biopsies) or (2) sebaceous hyperplasia without vellus involvement (13 biopsies). In my opinion, both may be correct as the pathophysiology can be a continuous process that starts with perifollicular inflammation leading to destruction of the vellus follicles and the elastic tissue around the follicular units (as published by Pirmez et al.) The retained sebaceous glands pop out through the devoid of elastic tissue skin easier (Figure 14.16)
- Other novel peculiar findings observed in 60 biopsies from FFA compared to 60 biopsies form AGA

included the following statistically significant results (Figure 14.17):
- Fat tissue infiltration at the isthmus level as clusters of cells or small globules in 70% (vs. 23% of the controls)
- Fat infiltration in the arrector pili muscle (APM) in 55% (vs. 15% of the controls)
- Sweat coils positioned in the reticular dermis in 43% (vs. 1.7% of the controls)

PEARLS

- FFA may co-exist with alopecia areata in the same patient and even in the same specimen (personal observation in 2 patients) (Figure 14.18)
- FFA shows epidermal and dermal atrophy in biopsies from the alopecic band in treatment-naïve patients (Saceda-Corralo et al.)

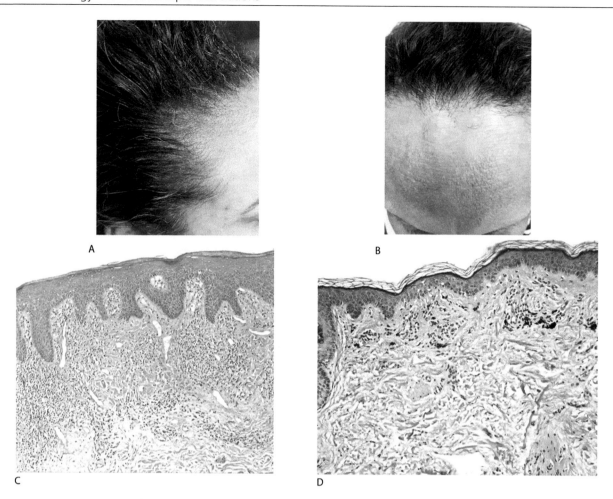

FIGURE 14.15 Pigmented contact dermatitis (A) is in the differential diagnosis of LPPigm (B). There is acanthosis, parakeratosis but minimal or no spongiosis, and patchy lichenoid infiltrate with melanophages in the dermis (C). In LPPigm (D), there is mild interface dermatitis with melanophages in perivascular and/or periadnexal distribution.

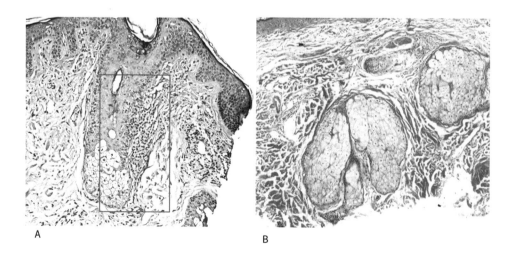

FIGURE 14.16 Two biopsies from facial papules reveal a continuum: (A) the inflammatory follicular pattern is supervened by the absence of follicles and only remaining sebaceous glands (B).

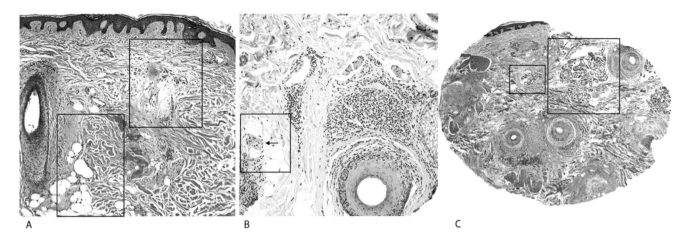

FIGURE 14.17 Fat tissue infiltration in the dermis at the level of the isthmus (A), in the arrector pili muscle (B) and sweat coils displacement at the level of the isthmus (C).

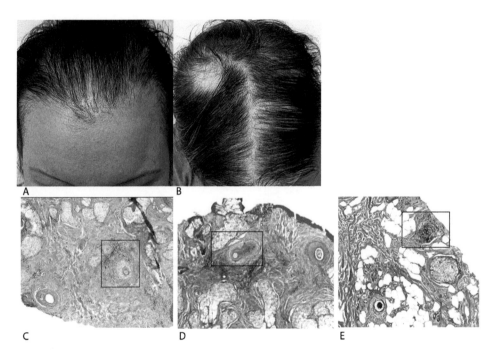

FIGURE 14.18 FFA and AA in the same patient (A, B). A biopsy from the frontal hairline shows features for both lymphocytic cicatricial alopecia (C, D) and swarm of bees for AA (E).

FURTHER READING

Anzai A, Pirmez R, Vincenzi C, Fabbrocini G, Romiti R, Tosti A. Trichoscopic findings of frontal fibrosing alopecia on the eyebrows: study of 151 cases. J Am Acad Dermatol. 2019 Dec 16.

Cervantes J, Miteva M. Distinct trichoscopic features of the sideburns in frontal fibrosing alopecia compared to the frontotemporal scalp. Skin Appendage Disord. 2018 Jan;4(1):50–4.

Chew AL, Bashir SJ, Wain EM, Fenton DA, Stefanato CM. Expanding the spectrum of frontal fibrosing alopecia: a unifying concept. J Am Acad Dermatol. 2010 Oct;63(4):653–60.

Donati A, Molina L, Doche I, Valente NS, Romiti R. Facial papules in frontal fibrosing alopecia: evidence of vellus follicle involvement. Arch Dermatol. 2011 Dec;147(12):1424–7.

Mervis JS, Borda LJ, Miteva M. Facial and extrafacial lesions in an ethnically diverse series of 91 patients with frontal fibrosing alopecia followed at a single center. Dermatology. 2019 235(2):112–9.

Miteva M, Castillo D, Sabiq S. Adipose infiltration of the dermis, involving the arrector pili muscle, and dermal displacement of eccrine sweat coils: new histologic observations in frontal fibrosing alopecia. Am J Dermatopathol. 2019 Jul;41(7):492–497.

Miteva M, Sabiq S. A new histologic pattern in 6 biopsies from early frontal fibrosing alopecia. Am J Dermatopathol. 2019 Feb;41(2):118–121.

Miteva M. Frontal fibrosing alopecia involving the limbs shows inflammatory pattern on histology: a review of 13 cases. Am J Dermatopathol. 2019 Aug 6.

Moreno-Arrones OM, Saceda-Corralo D, Fonda-Pascual P, Rodrigues-Barata AR, Buendia-Castano D, Alegre-Sanchez A, et al. Frontal fibrosing alopecia: clinical and prognostic classification. J Eur Acad Dermatol Venereol. 2017 Oct;31(10):1739–45.

Pedrosa AF, Duarte AF, Haneke E, Correia O. Yellow facial papules associated with frontal fibrosing alopecia: A distinct histologic pattern and response to isotretinoin. J Am Acad Dermatol. 2017 Oct;77(4):764–766.

Pirmez R, Barreto T, Duque-Estrada B, Quintella DC, Cuzzi T. Facial papules in frontal fibrosing alopecia: beyond vellus hair follicle involvement. Skin Appendage Disord. 2018 Aug;4(3):145–149.

Rossi A, Grassi S, Fortuna MC, Garelli V, Pranteda G, Caro G, et al. Unusual patterns of presentation of frontal fibrosing alopecia: a clinical and trichoscopic analysis of 98 patients. J Am Acad Dermatol. 2017 Jul;77(1):172–4.

Saceda-Corralo D, Desai K, Pindado-Ortega C, Moreno-Arrones OM, Vañó-Galván S, Miteva M. Histological evidence for epidermal and dermal atrophy of the alopecic band in treatment-naïve patients with frontal fibrosing alopecia. J Eur Acad Dermatol Venereol. 2021 Jan;35(1):e47–e49.

Fibrosing Alopecia in a Pattern Distribution

15

Contents

GENERAL CONCEPTS

Fibrosing alopecia in a pattern distribution (FAPD) was originally described by Zinkernagel and Trüeb as an unusual form of lichen planopilaris (LPP), showing concomitant miniaturization. It is unclear as to why the affected follicles attract immunologic lichenoid inflammation and initiate apoptosis-mediated process.

- This is a diffuse form of LPP in the area of typical male or female pattern hair loss but often some asymmetry of the affected area is present (personal communication with Dr. Maria Fernanda Gavazzoni) (Figure 15.1).
- Although women prevailed in the original case series (15 women and 4 men), men prevailed in our multicenter retrospective review of 26 cases (17 men and 9 women). A possible explanation may be the fact that men are usually not concerned about their common baldness and therefore FAPD can be missed in this group unless suspected and biopsied.
- FAPD can be associated with frontal fibrosing alopecia (FFA) and respectively eyebrow alopecia, limb alopecia and facial and extrafacial red dots.
- A clinical exam may miss the diagnosis although a close look revealing the pattern of "pink goose

bumps" in the patterned area, especially in the presence of dispersed ill-defined areas of atrichia, should suggest FAPD (Figure 15.2).
- Trichoscopy and histology are crucial for the diagnosis. *Trichoscopy* shows: (1) peripilar casts and interfollicular scale and erythema (Figures 15.3 and 15.4) and (2) single hairs or groups of hairs (2–4, "mini"-tufts) emerging from the same ostium in the area of thinning, surrounded by usually fine peripilar casts (Figure 15.4). These correspond to the compound follicles with perifollicular fibrosis and lichenoid inflammation.

MAIN HISTOLOGIC FEATURES

- Follicular miniaturization (terminal:vellus ratio is less than 2.2:1) (Figure 15.5).
- Perifollicular fibrosis and lichenoid inflammation affecting single terminal and vellus follicles and/or compound follicular structures (eyes and goggles) at the level of the upper follicle (Figures 15.6 and 15.7).
- Usually the features *are milder* that in classic LPP.
- Solar elastosis is prevalent in skin biopsies from FAPD as the diffuse thinning predisposes to actinic damage (Figure 15.5).

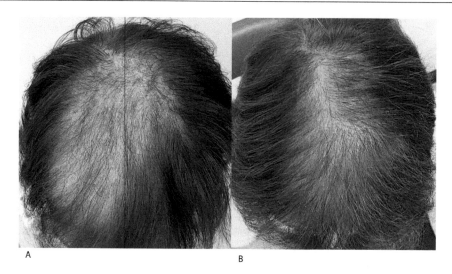

FIGURE 15.1   FAPD in a woman: (A) Before treatment; note the asymmetric outline of the affected area (the black line marks the middle). (B) After treatment with topical minoxidil, clobetasol and oral spironolactone).

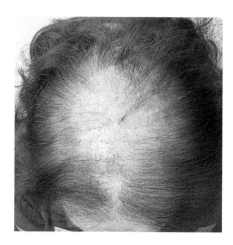

FIGURE 15.2   Another example of FAPD. Note the "pink goose bumps" on the clinical exam.

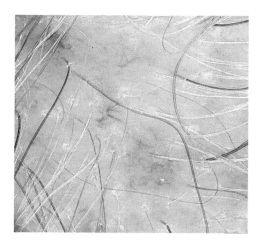

FIGURE 15.3   Dry trichoscopy shows loss of follicular openings, hair shaft variability and peripilar casts (×50).

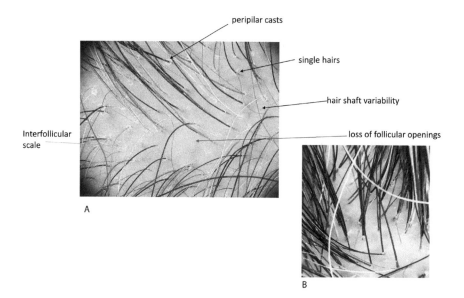

FIGURE 15.4   Other trichoscopic examples of FAPD reveal hair shaft variability and peripilar casts (A, ×50) and small tufts of hairs surrounded by peripilar casts (B, ×10, blue arrows).

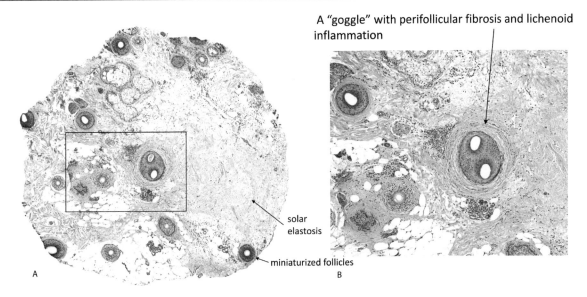

A "goggle" with perifollicular fibrosis and lichenoid inflammation

solar elastosis

miniaturized follicles

A

B

FIGURE 15.5   (A, B) There is significantly decreased follicular density with areas of follicular dropout, follicular miniaturization, compound follicular structures showing perifollicular fibrosis and lichenoid infiltrate; there is solar elastosis in the dermis.

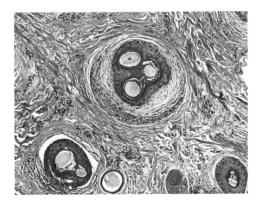

FIGURE 15.6   Perifollicular fibrosis and lichenoid inflammation surrounding compound follicles at the isthmus.

PEARLS

- In a patient with FFA, always look on the parietal scalp to exclude FAPD; in case of uncertainty – take a trichoscopy-guided biopsy.
- Distinguishing FAPD from AGA with perifollicular fibroplasia and inflammation ("complicated AGA") sometimes is not feasible and this should be noted in the report. As a rule, in FAPD there is an onion-like zone of pale/mucinous fibrosis and thinned follicular epithelium, lichenoid inflammation (vs. spongiosis with lymphocytic infiltrate in AGA (see Chapter 7).

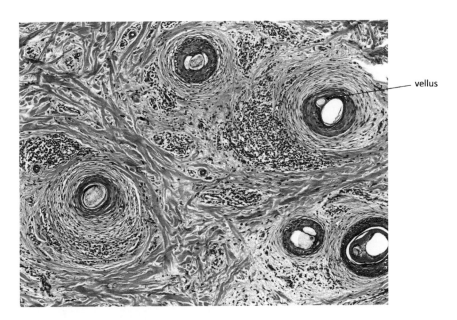

vellus

FIGURE 15.7   The perifollicular fibrosis and lichenoid inflammation affect single follicles or compound follicles, including vellus follicles.

FURTHER READING

Baquerizo Nole KL, Nusbaum B, Pinto GM, Miteva M. Lichen Planopilaris in the androgenetic alopecia area: a pitfall for hair transplantation. Skin Appendage Disord. 2015 Mar;1(1):49–53.

Zinkernagel MS, Trüeb RM. Fibrosing alopecia in a pattern distribution: patterned lichen planopilaris or androgenetic alopecia with a lichenoid tissue reaction pattern? Arch Dermatol. 2000;136:205–211.

Lupus Erythematosus of the Scalp

16

Contents

The most common type of hair loss in patients with systemic lupus erythematosus (SLE) is diffuse non-scarring alopecia consistent with telogen effluvium (see Chapter 10). Connective tissue diseases are associated with high levels of pro-inflammatory cytokines, which negatively impact the hair growth cycle leading to "inflammatory shedding". In this chapter, only specific presentations of lupus erythematosus associated alopecias are discussed.

DISCOID LUPUS ERYTHEMATOSUS

GENERAL CONCEPTS

Discoid lupus erythematosus (DLE) is the most common form of cutaneous lupus erythematosus and in 30–50% affects the scalp. It usually presents as well-demarcated, erythematous, scaly plaques with hair loss, atrophy, hyper- or hypopigmentation and follicular plugging (Figures 16.1 and 16.2). While in the early stage, the alopecia is non-scarring and some or even significant regrowth is possible, in 60% of the cases, DLE ultimately results in scarring alopecia. The following proposed criteria help distinguish DLE: (1) an erythematous to violaceous hue, (2) atrophic scarring and dyspigmentation, (3) follicular hyperkeratosis or plugging and (4) the presence of scarring alopecia. These changes, including telangiectasia, are more prominent in the center of the patch vs. the periphery in LPP and other scarring alopecias (Figure 16.3).

- Early cases may present as subtle lesions with hyperpigmentation only, particularly lacking atrophy and hair loss. We have described two cases of hyperpigmented patches mimicking pigmented lesions that have not eventuated in hair loss within the 5 years of observation (Figure 16.4). Similar large polycyclic hyperpigmented patches and scaly plaques involving the ventral abdomen has been reported in dogs with generalized discoid lupus erythematosus and correspond to prominent pigment incontinence in the biopsies.
- In linear presentation, the differential diagnosis includes linear lichen planopilaris (LPP) and morphea *en coup de sabre* (Figure 16.5).
- *Trichoscopy* shows follicular red dots (Figure 16.6), which are considered specific for DLE, large irregular yellow dots with arborizing vessels (red spider over a yellow dot) (Figure 16.6), monstrous vessels (Figure 16.3), blue-gray dots in a speckled pattern

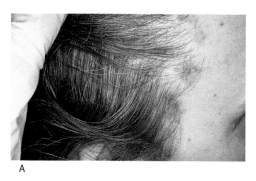
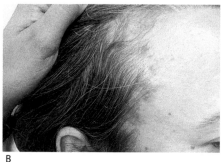

FIGURE 16.1   Discoid lupus erythematosus involving the hairline mimicking seborrheic dermatitis (A—before, and B—after treatment).

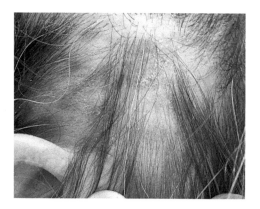

FIGURE 16.2   Erythematous scaly plaques in another case of discoid lupus erythematosus.

(see Chapter 13), interfollicular scale and follicular keratotic plugs (Figure 16.6). In dark skin, blue-white veil-like features can be appreciated that correspond to the combination of epidermal hyperkeratosis and prominent pigment incontinence at the dermo-epidermal junction. The above-mentioned features are all good sites to take the scalp biopsy from, particularly the keratotic plugs.

Main Histologic Features

- Both horizontal and vertical sections are useful to make the diagnosis.
- On vertical sections, there are classic findings of interface dermatitis (vacuolar degeneration) involving the dermo-epidermal junction, thickened basement membrane, periadnexal lymphoid cell infiltrate and mucin in the dermis and subdermis in a diffuse pattern (vs. perifollicular pattern in LPP). The epidermis shows atrophy or atrophy alternating with hyperplasia (Figure 16.7).

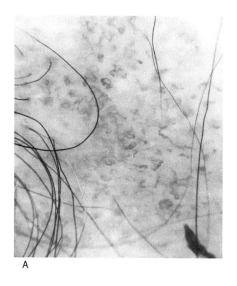
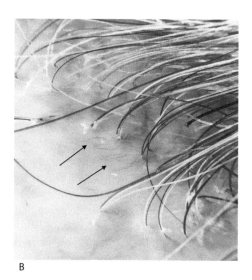

FIGURE 16.3   (A) Monstrous (thick arborizing vessels) are prominent in the center of the alopecic patch in DLE and correspond to prominent dilated capillaries on histology (see Figure 16.6). (B) In LPP, there are linear vessels at the rim of the alopecic patch.

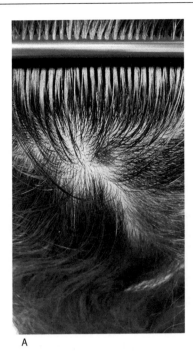

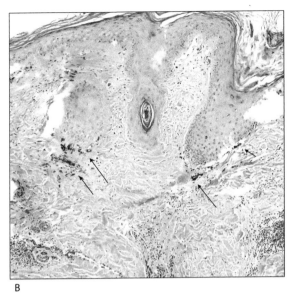

B

FIGURE 16.4 (A) Discoid lupus erythematosus, biopsy proven, presenting as brown patches. (B) There is prominent pigment incontinence on histology.

- On horizontal sections, the main features include interface dermatitis and thickened basement membrane involving the follicular epithelium, pigment incontinence and absent sebaceous glands (Figure 16.8).
- The follicular infundibula are plugged by keratin (Figure 16.6).

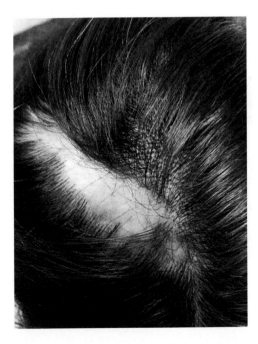

FIGURE 16.5 Linear DLE mimicking linear morphea *en coup de sabre.*

- The lymphocytic infiltrate extends along the follicular epithelium and the eccrine glands, as well as in a perivascular pattern with red blood cells extravasation in the early cases (corresponding to the follicular red dots) (Figure 16.9).
- There are lymphoid follicles (germinal center like-collections) of lymphocytes and plasmacytoid cells in the subdermis (Figure 16.9).
- Two patterns have been recognized on pathology in horizontal sections: (1) alopecia areata (AA)-like pattern with basaloid aggregates of follicular epithelium, deep perifollicular inflammation, pigmented casts and increased catagen/telogen count and (2) LPP-like pattern with perifollicular lamellar fibrosis and moderate perifollicular lymphocytic inflammation at the isthmus and infundibular level (Figure 16.10). In my opinion, the AA-like pattern is more common in early DLE biopsies.

LUPUS PROFUNDUS (LUPUS PANNICULITIS)

GENERAL CONCEPTS

Lupus profundus/Lupus panniculitis (LPr) is a rare variant of cutaneous lupus erythematosus that primarily involves the deep dermis and adipose tissue as lobular panniculitis with

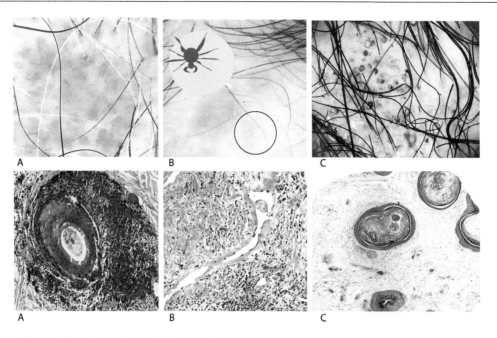

FIGURE 16.6   Follicular red dots (A, x10), irregular large yellow dots with arborizing vessels (B, x10) and keratotic plugs (C, x20) with their histologic correlates.

lymphocytic infiltration and hyaline fat necrosis. On the scalp, it most commonly presents as linear scarring alopecia along the Blaschko's lines but annular, patch-like (Figure 16.11) and ulcerated lesions are also possible.

- On *trichoscopy*, there is absence of dermo-epidermal junctional involvement and keratotic plugs as in DLE. There can be a diffuse erythema with violaceous hue of the skin, large yellow dots and monstrous vessels (Figure 16.11).

- *Linear and annular lupus panniculitis of the scalp (LALPS)* is a unique subset of LPr, which results in non-scarring alopecia along the Blaschko's lines of the scalp in young East Asian men. It presents as annular or weirdly configured patches with or without erythema. Compared to classic LPr, this form has a reversible clinical course, and fewer associations with SLE.

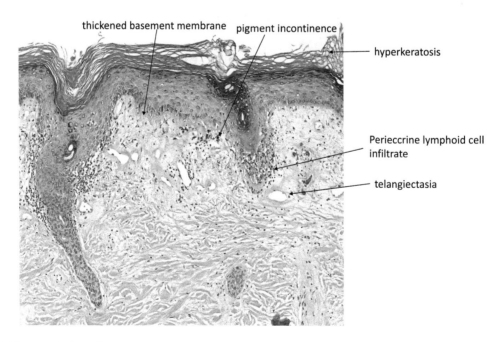

FIGURE 16.7   DLE on vertical sections.

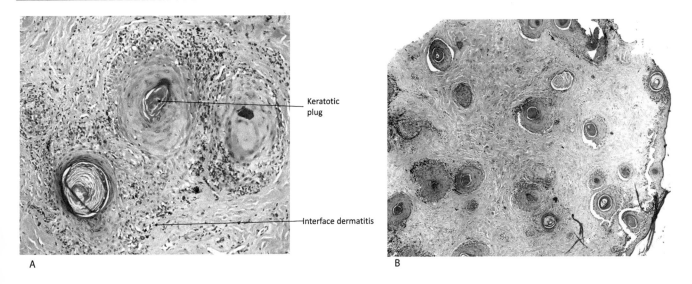

FIGURE 16.8 (A, B) Interface dermatitis with pigment incontinence involving the follicular epithelium at the upper follicular level. Note the keratotic plugs.

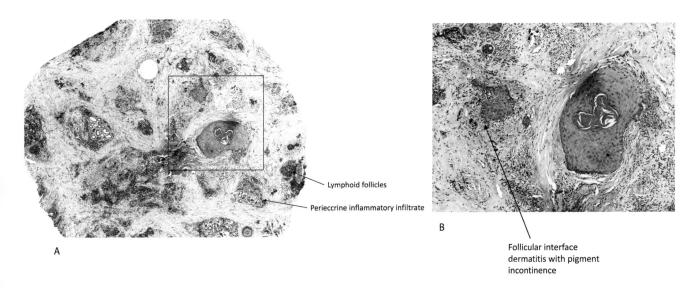

FIGURE 16.9 (A, B) Another example of DLE on horizontal sections.

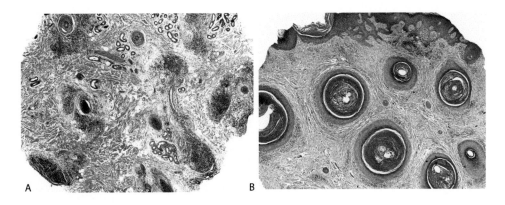

FIGURE 16.10 Alopecia areata-like pattern in DLE (A) and LPP-like pattern in DLE (B).

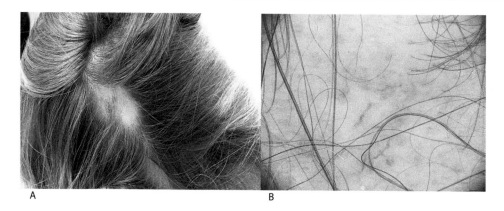

FIGURE 16.11 (A) Lupus profundus presenting as patches mimicking alopecia areata. (B) On trichoscopy, there are irregular yellow dots and monstrous vessels. Note the absence of keratotic plugs (×40).

MAIN HISTOLOGIC FEATURES (Figures 16.12 and 16.13)

- Lymphocytes and plasma cells rim the fat cells in the lobules (but also can be found in the septa and in the dermis); nuclear fragmentation can be noted
- Lymphoid follicles
- Hyalinization of the fat
- Deposition of mucin in the subdermis
- Presence of interface dermatitis, periadnexal infiltrate and mucin deposition in the dermis are also possible

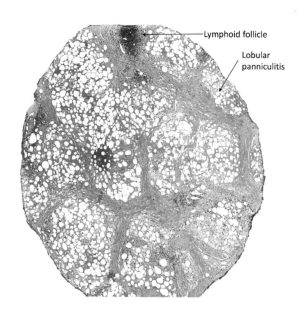

FIGURE 16.12 Lupus profundus of the scalp on horizontal sections.

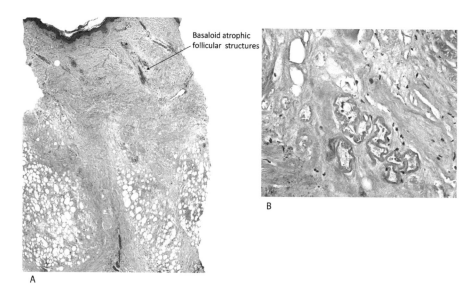

FIGURE 16.13 (A, B) Lupus profundus of the scalp on vertical sections. The hyaline fat necrosis is shown on higher magnification on (B).

NON-SCARRING ALOPECIA IN SYSTEMIC LUPUS ERYTHEMATOSUS

The non-scarring alopecia in SLE usually indicates an active disease. It can present as mild or severe diffuse alopecia (the majority of the cases) or as localized alopecic patches (Figure 16.14). In fact, non-scarring alopecia is now part of the new proposed criteria in the American College of Rheumatology classification criteria for SLE. The patchy subtype has been previously misdiagnosed as alopecia areata but now is considered a specific form of alopecia restricted to

with germinal center-like lymphoid follicles is the main finding (Figures 16.15 and 16.16). Keratotic plugs are missing, the epidermis is usually atrophic and the sebaceous glands are preserved (in comparison to DLE). Chanprapaph et al. showed recently interface changes along the dermo-epidermal junction in 87.5% of the 32 biopsies and vacuolar changes along the follicular epithelium in 40.6%. Interestingly, none had basement membrane thickening. Horizontal sections showed decreased follicular density (average 17.6) and increased percentage of catagen/telogen follicles (average 16.7).

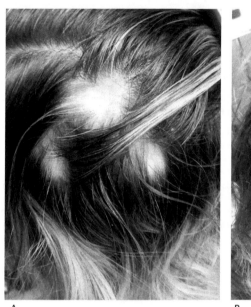 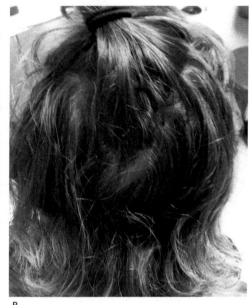

A   B

FIGURE 16.14 Non-scarring patchy alopecia in SLE: (A) before and (B) after treatment.

patients with SLE. This type of hair loss is possibly related to local vasculitis and has the potential for complete regrowth with immunomodulatory treatment. It presents usually with decreased hair density (rather than complete hair loss) and erythema in the patches. It has been shown to correlate with higher SLE Disease Activity Index 2000 score and proteinuria (more than 1g/d).

- *Trichoscopy* does not show black dots and broken hairs vs. AA. There are arborizing vessels and thin hypopigmented hairs.

MAIN HISTOLOGIC FEATURES

- In my experience, pronounced interface dermatitis with dermal mucin deposition, periadnexal infiltrate

PEARLS

- The pattern of mucin deposition is diffuse, superficial and deep in DLE vs. folliculocentric as perifollicular mucinous fibrosis in LPP.
- There is no peribulbar infiltrate in the AA-like subtype of DLE vs. AA.
- The lupus band test from lesional skin shows granular deposition of immunoglobulin and complement at the dermo-epidermal junction in over 80% of the specimens with DLE.
- Hyalinization of the fat can be observed in any scalp biopsies from patients with SLE.
- CD123 positive plasmocytoid dendritic cells (PDC) have been shown arranged in clusters in the perivascular, perieccrine and perifollicular infiltrate in DLE vs. mainly arranged as single, interstitial cell in LPP or central centrifugal cicatricial alopecia.
- DLE can be associated with frontal fibrosing alopecia.

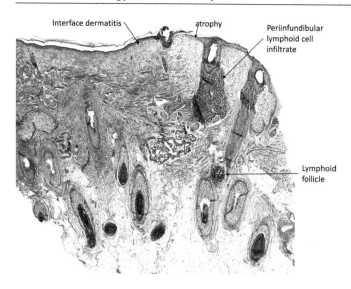

Interface dermatitis   atrophy   Periinfundibular lymphoid cell infiltrate

Lymphoid follicle

FIGURE 16.15   Non-scarring diffuse alopecia in SLE on vertical sections.

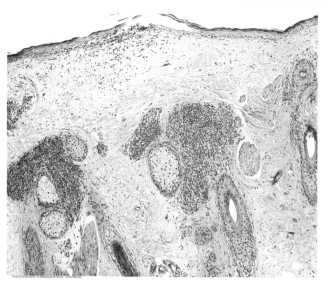

FIGURE 16.16   Non-scarring diffuse alopecia in SLE showing the pronounced interface dermatitis and dense perivascular and periadnexal lymphoid cell infiltrate. Note the presence of sebaceous glands.

FURTHER READING

Chanprapaph K, Udompanich S, Visessiri Y, Ngamjanyaporn P, Suchonwanit P. Nonscarring alopecia in systemic lupus erythematosus: a cross-sectional study with trichoscopic, histopathologic, and immunopathologic analyses. J Am Acad Dermatol. 2019 Dec;81(6):1319–29.

Concha JSS, Werth VP. Alopecias in lupus erythematosus. Lupus Sci Med. 2018 Oct 25;5(1):e000291.doi: 10.1136/lupus-2018-000291

Elman SA, Joyce C, Nyberg F, et al. Development of classification criteria for discoid lupus erythematosus: results of a delphi exercise. J Am Acad Dermatol 2017;77:261–7.

Fening K, Parekh V, McKay K. CD123 immunohistochemistry for plasmacytoid dendritic cells is useful in the diagnosis of scarring alopecia. J Cutan Pathol. 2016 Aug;43(8):643–8.

Lueangarun S, Subpayasarn U, Tempark T. Distinctive lupus panniculitis of scalp with linear alopecia along Blaschko's lines: a review of the literature. Int J Dermatol. 2019 Feb;58(2):144–50.

Olivry T, Linder KE, Banovic F. Cutaneous lupus erythematosus in dogs: a comprehensive review. BMC Vet Res. 2018 Apr 18; 14(1):132.

Trüeb RM. Involvement of scalp and nails in lupus erythematosus. Lupus. 2010 Aug;19(9):1078–86.

Udompanich S, Chanprapaph K, Suchonwanit P. Linear and annular lupus panniculitis of the scalp: case report with emphasis on trichoscopic findings and review of the literature. Case Rep Dermatol. 2019 Jun 6;11(2):157–65.

Traction Alopecia

17

Contents

GENERAL CONCEPTS

Traction alopecia (TA) results from the use of high-tension hairstyles. The extent and the duration of the pulling forces increase the risk of irreversible TA.

- It is most common in African American women (30%).
- The frequent use of tight buns or ponytails, the attachment of weaves or hair extensions and tight braids (such as cornrows and dreadlocks) are the highest-risk hairstyles for irreversible TA.
- Chemical relaxation is an additional risk factor.
- Patients may report tenderness, paresthesias and headache.
- The hair loss can occur at any area depending on the configuration of the hairstyle and the bulk of the pressure induced, but it is most common on frontal and temporal scalp and less common on the vertex and occipital scalp.
- The clinical pattern can be *marginal traction alopecia* (a band-like alopecia along the margins of the fronto-temporal scalp and the temples that leave a margin of vellus hairs marking the preexisting hairline known as "fringe sign") (Figure 17.1) and *non-marginal traction alopecia*: patches throughout the scalp at the site of installment of the hairstyles with tension such as micro-braids or cornrows (Figure 17.2A–C).

ACUTE TRACTION ALOPECIA

- Acute TA is reversible and regrowth can be expected within 6 months if the offensive tension on the hairs is removed.
- In the early stage, patients present with patches of non-scarring hair loss along the area of the scalp that has undergone excessive tension over short time. The patches may mimic alopecia areata or trichotillomania (Figure 17.3).

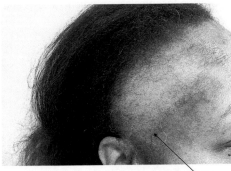

Fringe sign

FIGURE 17.1 Marginal traction alopecia showing vellus hairs retained in a band-like fashion at the edge of the hairline.

119

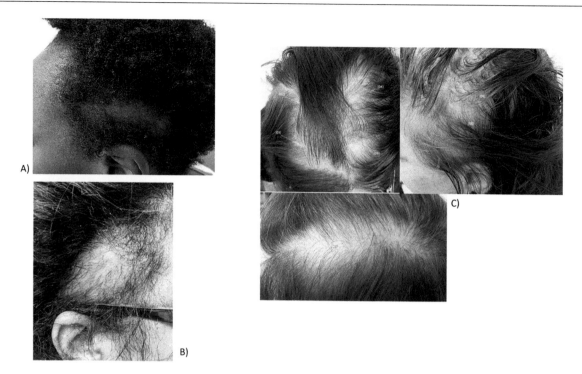

FIGURE 17.2   Three cases of non-marginal traction alopecia showing one (A, B) and numerous ill-defined patches (C) at the site of installment of the braids.

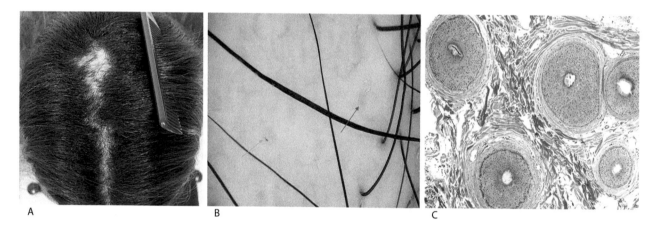

FIGURE 17.3   Acute traction alopecia: (A) A patch on vertex at the site of installment of a tight weave. The patient experienced pain and removed the weave after 3 days. (B) On trichoscopy, there are yellow dots and a broken (flame-like) hair (×40). (C) On histology, this corresponds to trichomalacia, pigmented casts and catagen/telogen shift.

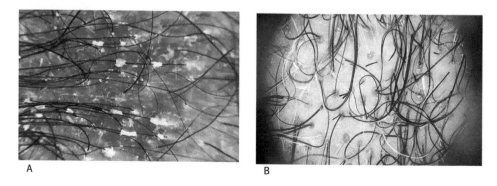

FIGURE 17.4   Two more examples of acute TA: hair casts encircle the proximal portions of the hair shafts in marginal TA in a young girl who had abrupt hair loss after wearing a very tight ponytail for days (A). Broken hairs at different levels are noted in the frontal scalp after a glued wig has been removed in another woman (B, ×20).

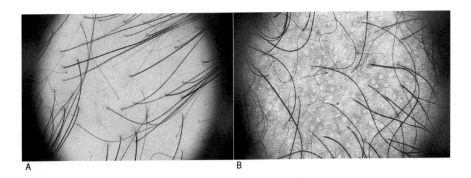

FIGURE 17.5 Chronic TA. (A) The trichoscopic image was obtained from the patient in Figure 17.2 (C): note the loss of follicular openings and increased number of thin hairs (×20). The trichoscopic image on the left was obtained from the patient in Figure 17.2 (A): note the loss of follicular openings (red arrows), pinpoint white dots (blue arrows) and prevalent thin hairs (×20).

CHRONIC (LATE) TRACTION ALOPECIA

If the traumatic hairstyling continues without appropriate intervention, the hair loss will progress to irreversible scarring alopecia.

- On *trichoscopy,* there are black dots and broken hairs. Broken hairs at different levels and follicular pustules are often a clue to acute traumatic injury (Figure 17.4). Yellow dots can be seen in skin types I-III and correspond to empty follicular openings (Figure 17.3). Hair casts (white or yellowish cylinders that encircle the proximal emergence of the affected terminal hair shafts) are a sign of ongoing traction and therefore most numerous at the margin of the alopecic area (Figure 17.4). They slide easily and correspond to the desquamated inner or outer root sheath. In chronic TA, there are less hair casts and there is loss of follicular openings (follicular dropout) with vellus hairs prevailing over terminal hairs (Figure 17.5).

MAIN HISTOLOGIC FEATURES

- Acute TA shows features similar to trichotillomania:
  - Reduced hair density with increased catagen/telogen count (that correspond to the traumatized hairs) (Figure 17.6). Absence of swarm of bees lymphocytic infiltrate is a clue to acute TA vs. AA
  - Trichomalacia (distorted hair shafts) and pigmented casts can be noted (see also Traumatic Alopecia)

- Chronic TA shows features for non-inflammatory scarring alopecia:

  - Decreased total number of follicles
  - Follicular dropout (fibrotic tracts replacing entire follicular units): in TA, usually all terminal hairs from a single unit are pulled out) (Figures 17.7 and 17.8)

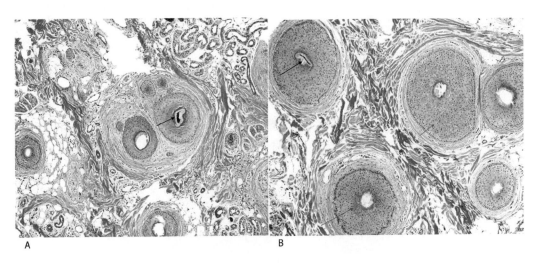

FIGURE 17.6 (A) Acute traction alopecia (the biopsy was obtained from the patient on Figure 17.3): zip sign (black arrow), (B) catagen follicles (red arrows point to increased apoptosis in the outer root sheath), and absence of hair shafts (due to abrupt extraction by the pulling forces [blue arrow]).

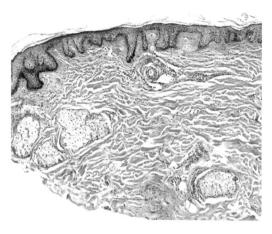

FIGURE 17.7   Traction alopecia (vertical section): there are follicular dropout (red arrow), preserved sebaceous glands and single vellus follicles.

- Preservation of the sebaceous glands and follicular units composed only of sebaceous glands) (Figures 17.8 and 17.9)
- The vellus follicles outnumber the terminal follicles (decreased terminal:vellus ratio)
- Fragmented hair shafts (Figure 17.10)

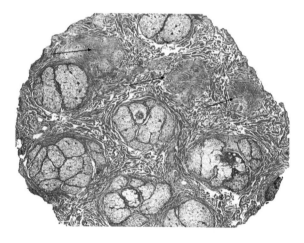

FIGURE 17.8   Chronic TA: the available follicular units contain only sebaceous glands. There is follicular dropout (black arrows).

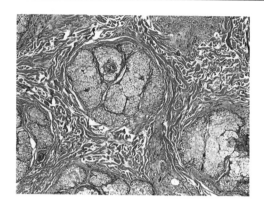

FIGURE 17.9   A high power view of the follicular units containing only intact sebaceous glands in chronic TA.

PEARLS

- Presence of "goggle-like" compound follicular structures and only focal preservation of the sebaceous glands is a clue to central centrifugal cicatricial alopecia (both diagnoses coincide in many cases).

FURTHER READING

Billero V, Miteva M. Traction alopecia: the root of the problem. Clin Cosmet Investig Dermatol. 2018 Apr 6;11:149–159.

Goldberg LJ. Cicatricial marginal alopecia: is it all traction? Br J Dermatol. 2009 Jan;160(1):62–8.

Miteva M, Tosti A. 'A detective look' at hair biopsies from African American patients. Br Dermatol. 2012 Jun;166(6):1289–94.

Samrao A, Price VH, Zedek D, Mirmirani P. The "Fringe Sign"—A useful clinical finding in traction alopecia of the marginal hairline. Dermatol Online J. 2011 Nov 15;17(11):1.

Tosti A, Miteva M, Torres F, Vincenzi C, Romanelli P. Hair casts are a dermoscopic clue for the diagnosis of traction alopecia. Br J Dermatol. 2010 Dec;163(6):1353–5.

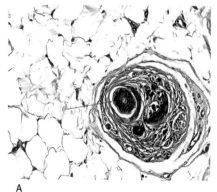
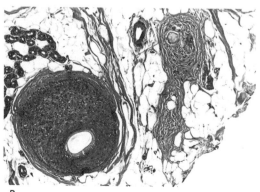

A   B

FIGURE 17.10   (A, B) Fragmented hair shafts within fibrous streamers in TA.

Central Centrifugal Cicatricial Alopecia (CCCA)

18

Contents

GENERAL CONCEPTS

Central centrifugal cicatricial alopecia (CCCA) is the most common cicatricial alopecia in African American women. It is characterized by chronic and progressive central scalp hair loss, which starts on the crown and spreads peripherally but spares the lateral, frontal and posterior scalp (Figure 18.1). Advanced cases show a smooth and shiny scalp (Figure 18.2).

- There might be slight erythema and grouping of 2–3 hairs coming out of one follicle (polytrichia). Symptoms can range from none to soreness, itching and burning.
- Hair breakage on the vertex has been reported as a possible early clinical presentation of CCCA that has been confirmed on pathology (Figure 18.3).
- Early cases are difficult to distinguish from androgenetic alopecia and pathology is very important to make the diagnosis (Figures 18.1 and 18.4).
- CCCA can present as "patchy"-interconnected alopecic patches with a maze-like appearance in the occipital and parietal scalp (Figure 18.5).
- Small series have shown that CCCA can be inherited in an autosomal dominant fashion, with a partial penetrance and a strong modifying effect of hairstyling and sex.
- Upregulation of genes implicated in fibroproliferative disorders (platelet-derived growth factor gene [PDGF], collagen I gene [COL I], collagen III gene [COL III], matrix metallopeptidase 1 gene [MMP1], matrix metallopeptidase 2 gene [MMP2], matrix metallopeptidase 7 gene [MMP7] and matrix metallopeptidase 9 gene [MMP9]) has been detected in patients with CCCA.
- Prevalence of *PADI3* mutation was higher among patients with CCCA than in a control cohort of women of African ancestry according to a recent exome sequencing study.
- CCCA has been described in teenage children, which adds weight to the concept that genetic susceptibility may play a significant role in the pathogenesis.
- On *trichoscopy*, the most common features are: (1) the peripilar gray/white halo that is a specific and sensitive dermatoscopic sign for CCCA (Figure 18.6, see also Chapter 5); (2) irregular honeycomb-pigmented network that represents the hyperpigmented rete ridges and the hypomelanotic dermal papillae (Figure 18.6); (3) irregularly distributed pinpoint white dots (Figure 18.7); (4) hair shaft variability that corresponds to the decreased terminal:vellus ratio observed on histology (Figure 18.7) and (5) white patches that represent follicular dropout (Figure 18.8). Less frequent are perifollicular and interfollicular scales that should not be mistaken for peripilar casts since the latter are tightly attached tubular structures that encircle the proximal portion of the hair shafts, and individual black dots or broken hairs. Of note, there are no peripilar casts in CCCA (Figure 18.9).

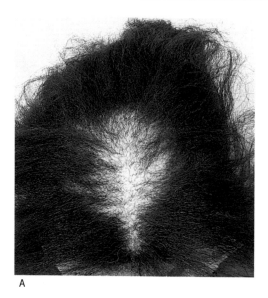
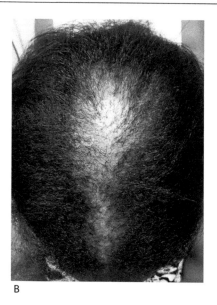

FIGURE 18.1   (A, B) Hair loss involving the crown and vertex that spreads peripherally but spares the lateral, frontal and posterior scalp is typical for central centrifugal cicatricial alopecia.

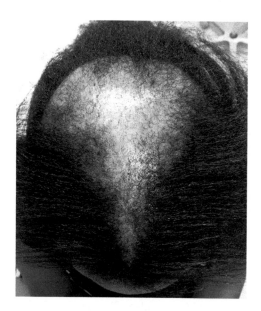

FIGURE 18.2   Central centrifugal cicatricial alopecia; note the smooth and shiny scalp in a more advanced case.

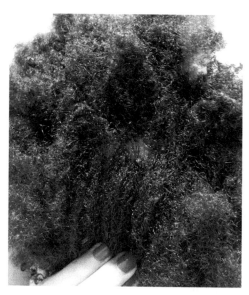

FIGURE 18.3   This young patient has no clear patches of hair loss but complaints of hair breakage on the central scalp, which led to the diagnosis of CCCA on histology.

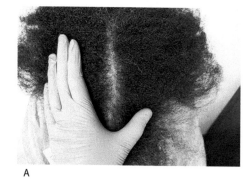
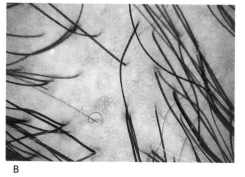

FIGURE 18.4   (A) This case of androgenetic alopecia demonstrates clinical similarity to CCCA. (B) Trichoscopy shows irregular pigmented network and hair shaft variability, which indicates towards AGA (×40). However, in such cases a biopsy is necessary to confirm the diagnosis.

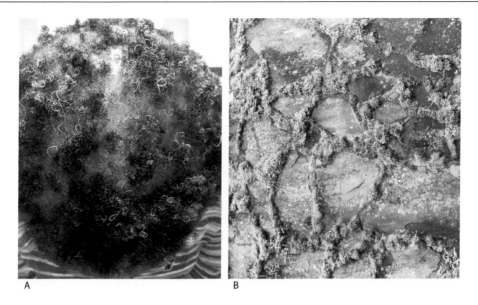

FIGURE 18.5   (A) Patchy CCCA presents with a pattern of hairless areas among preserved islands of hair resembling (B) a maze-like growth of moss on a stone; this type involves also the parietal and occipital scalp.

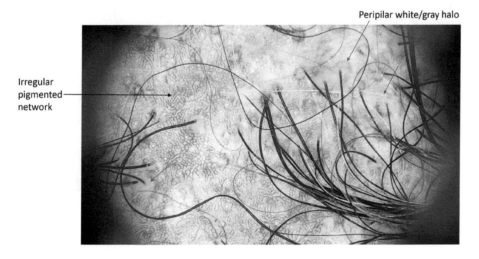

FIGURE 18.6   Loss of follicular openings, irregular pigmented network and peripilar white/gray halo are typical features on trichoscopy of CCCA (×40).

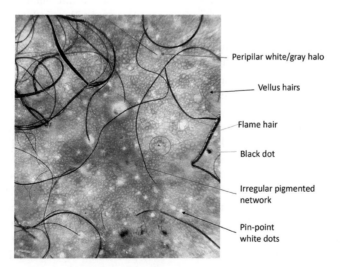

FIGURE 18.7   Irregular distribution of pinpoint white dots, irregular pigmented network, peripilar white/gray halo, black dots and a broken hair (flame hair) in CCCA. Note also the hair shaft variability (×20).

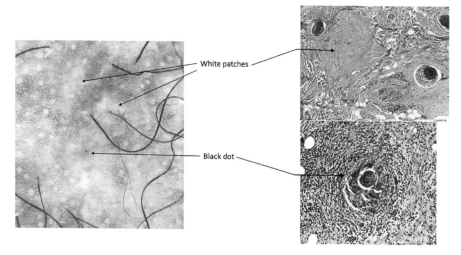

FIGURE 18.8 White patches in CCCA correspond to areas of follicular dropout and black dots correspond to the destroyed hair follicle (×20).

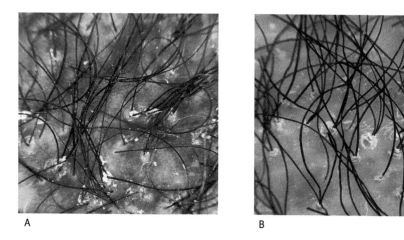

A   B

FIGURE 18.9 The distinction between perifollicular and interfollicular scaling in (A) CCCA and (B) peripilar casts in lichen planopilaris (×20).

MAIN HISTOLOGIC FEATURES

- Horizontal sections are optimal for the diagnosis since they allow for assessment of the follicular architecture and for identification of a focal disease. There is altered follicular architecture with decreased follicular density and ultimate loss of the follicular units (follicular dropout) (Figure 18.10).
- The sebaceous glands are usually absent or diminished. It is not uncommon to detect focal preservation of the sebaceous lobules surrounding a vellus follicle in "a hug" (Figures 18.10 and 18.11).
- In the active stages, there could be follicular lichenoid inflammation but it is uncommon to see pronounced lichenoid infiltrate and follicular apoptosis compared to lichen planopilaris; in the later stages, concentric onion-like follicular fibrosis is the main feature (Figures 18.10 and 18.11).

- "Goggle"-like structures, which occur due to fusion of the outer root sheaths of adjacent follicles entrapped in inflammation and concentric fibrosis (Figures 18.12 and 18.13).
- Premature desquamation of the inner root sheath (IRS) – individual or compound follicular structures surrounded by perifollicular fibrosis detected not only in affected but also in unaffected follicles (Figure 18.10).
- Lamellar hyperkeratosis/parakeratosis in the hair canal, which occurs likely as a reaction to follicular trauma in the hair follicle that has prematurely shed the IRS (Figure 18.14).
- Fragmented hair shafts in the dermis by themselves or in granulomas are a common finding (Figure 18.15).
- Follicular miniaturization of about 2:1 (decreased terminal:vellus ratio)
- Dilated syringoma-like eccrine ducts are not uncommon but they are not specific and can be encountered in lichen panopilaris (Figure 18.16).

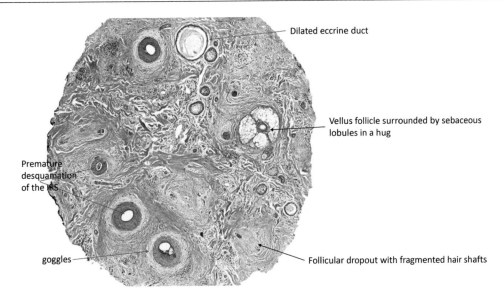

FIGURE 18.10   A classic example of CCCA in a horizontal section (isthmus level).

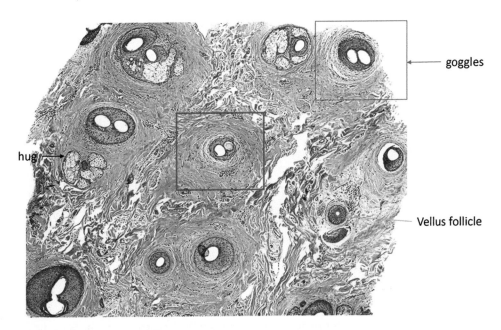

FIGURE 18.11   Another example of CCCA in horizontal sections demonstrating goggles and only focal preservation of the sebaceous lobules.

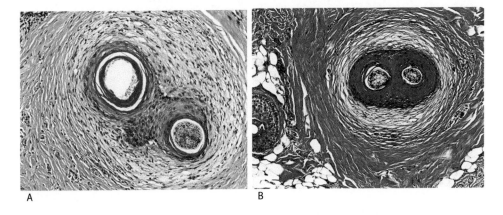

FIGURE 18.12   (A, B) Goggles (two follicles connected by the fusion of their outer root sheaths) are surrounded by concentric fibrosis. Note the absence of inner root sheath.

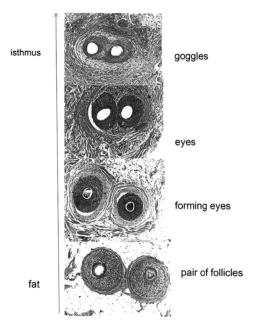

isthmus

goggles

eyes

forming eyes

pair of follicles

fat

FIGURE 18.13 In CCCA, the goggles form "through" eyes.

PEARLS

- If peripilar casts are found on trichoscopy, the diagnosis of CCCA should be re-considered to lichen planopilaris (LPP) or fibrosing alopecia in a pattern distribution (FAPD).
- Melanophages that appear spindled and slender are not uncommon in the upper dermis in various amounts from a few random cells to clusters of cells, and should not be overcalled a melanocytic nevus by the morphologic similarity to nevus cells; there is a lack of dermal sclerosis (Figure 18.17) (personal observation). This may contribute to the variations in the color intensity of the irregular pigmented network in the same scalp.
- The absence of follicular apoptosis and only mild/absent lichenoid inflammation favors CCCA over lichen planopilaris.
- Histologic clues pointing to ethnicity in horizontal sections of scalp biopsies are reviewed in Chapter 6.
- Early-stage CCCA that presents with hair thining may be mistaken for AGA, if a biopsy is not taken.

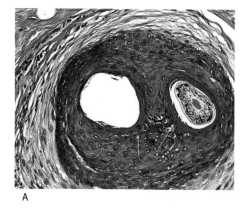

A

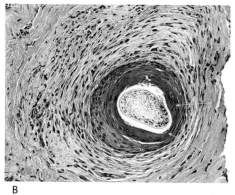

B

FIGURE 18.14 (A, B) Lamellar parakeratosis or hyperkeratosis lines up the follicular canal where the IRS is missing. The parakeratosis may be regarded as sign of follicular trauma occurring at the sites of geometric weakness along the follicle.

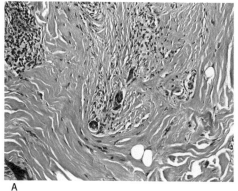

A

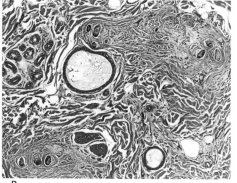

B

FIGURE 18.15 (A, B) Fragmented hair shafts from the destructed hair follicles lie individually or in clusters in the dermis surrounded by granulomatous inflammation.

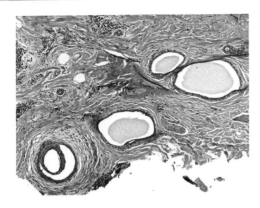

FIGURE 18.16 Prominent syringoma-like dilated eccrine ducts in CCCA are not specific and can be encountered in other scarring alopecias; note the premature desquamation of the IRS in the follicle.

FURTHER READING

Aguh C, Dina Y, Talbot CC Jr, Garza L. Fibroproliferative genes are preferentially expressed in central centrifugal cicatricial alopecia. J Am Acad Dermatol. 2018 Nov;79(5):904–12.e1.

Eginli AN, Dlova NC, McMichael A. Central centrifugal cicatricial alopecia in children: a case series and review of the literature. Pediatr Dermatol. 2017 Mar;34(2):133–7.

Malki L, Sarig O, Romano MT, Méchin MC, Peled A, Pavlovsky M, Warshauer E, Samuelov L, Uwakwe L, Briskin V, Mohamad J, Gat A, Isakov O, Rabinowitz T, Shomron N, Adir N, Simon M, McMichael A, Dlova NC, Betz RC, Sprecher E. Variant PADI3 in central centrifugal cicatricial alopecia. N Engl J Med. 2019 Feb 28;380(9):833–41.

Miteva M, Tosti A. 'A detective look' at hair biopsies from African American patients. Br J Dermatol. 2012 Jun;166(6):1289–94.

Miteva M, Tosti A. Pathologic diagnosis of central centrifugal cicatricial alopecia on horizontal sections. Am J Dermatopathol. 2014 Nov;36(11):859–64; quiz 865–7.

Olsen EA, Callender V, Sperling L, et al. Central scalp alopecia photographic scale in African American women. Dermatol Ther 2008;21:264–7.

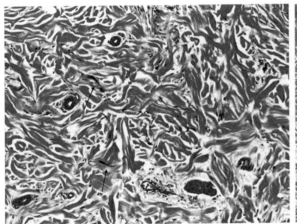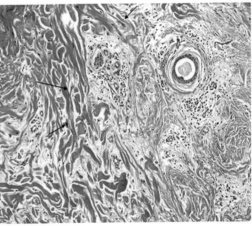

FIGURE 18.17 In my experience, dendritic melanophages are seen in at least 1 out of 3 CCCA cases in various proportions from very few to clusters mimicking the histologic pattern in a common blue nevus.

Folliculitis Decalvans

19

Contents

GENERAL CONCEPTS

Folliculitis decalvans (FD) is a neutrophilic primary cicatricial alopecia characterized by chronic inflammation, hair tufting and follicular destruction leading to irreversible hair loss and permanent scarring of the scalp.

- Clinically FD presents with (1) *typical pattern*: follicular papules and pustules, erythema, hyperkeratosis and prominent tufting (more than 6 hairs emerging from the same ostia), yellow crusts (Figure 19.1) and (2) concomitant presence of features for both FD and lichen planopilaris (LPP): *folliculitis decalvans lichen planopilaris phenotypic spectrum (FDLPPPS)* (Figure 19.2) (see also Chapter 13). These two patterns are considered by some authors rather a continuum in the evolution of the lesions starting with more acute type of neutrophilic inflammation at the beginning (typical FD) that evolves into chronic lympho-plasmocytic chronic inflammation, which is often recalcitrant to a monotherapy with an antibacterial agent and requires anti-inflammatory/immunomodulatory treatment (FDLPPPS).
- The pathogenesis is unclear but it has been centered on the isolation *S. aureus* from FD lesions. Therefore, the mainstay therapy includes antimicrobial treatment, which leads to clinical remission; however, recurrence is common. The dysbiosis of microbiota in the hair follicle that triggers normal immune host cell response pushes the immune system response into overdrive, exposing follicular neo-antigens and promoting ongoing and chronic abnormal immune response. However, a recent work showed that statistically significant *S. aureus* levels are found in patients with a typical FD pattern compared to patients with FDLPPPS (*S. aureus* levels were higher than 20% in the typical FD pattern whereas they were less than 20% in the FDLPPPS by using the linear discriminant analysis effect size tool), which questions the real impact of *S. aureus* in the pathogenesis of FD, particularly in the FDLPPPS subtype.
- Tufted folliculitis (TF) is considered by some authors analogous with FD; however, it is rather a morphologic term for fibrosis-induced gathering of adjacent follicular structures as it is a feature of several scarring alopecias including LPP, central centrifugal cicatricial alopecia, and acne keloidalis nuchae. However, the area of tufting involved in these conditions is usually focal vs. more uniform involvement in FD and the tufts are usually composed of 2–4 follicles (mini-tufts).
- Lesions are located on the vertex and occipital scalp and are often symptomatic with itch, trichodynia, burning and pain, which often correspond to florid local inflammation on histology.
- Late-stage FD is characterized by scarred areas of various extent with shiny flesh-colored surface and irreversible tufts, which are of aesthetic concern (a curious observation is that the hairs in the tufts demonstrate continuous growth with the rest of the hair (Figure 19.1), which contradicts

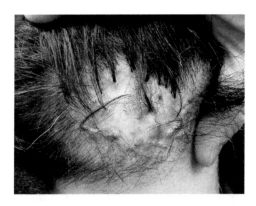

FIGURE 19.1 Typical pattern of folliculitis decalvans: erythematous papules and tufts of hairs (polytrichia) with scarring alopecia on the occipital scalp.

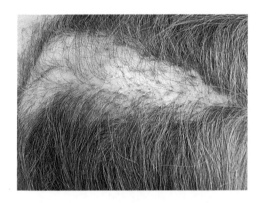

FIGURE 19.2 Lichen planopilaris folliculitis decalvans phenotypic spectrum (LPPFDPS): a large area of cicatricial alopecia on the vertex with erythematous papules, hyperkeratosis, yellow scale crusts and less prominent tufts.

the original concept that the tufting of hair is partially caused by retention of telogen hairs within the involved follicular units).

- On *trichoscopy,* the most common finding is (1) tufts of hairs (more than 6) which correspond to the compound follicular structures of several follicular infundibula joined by the their outer root sheaths and surrounded by fibrosis (Figure 19.3); (2) at the emergence base, the tufts are surrounded by prominent yellow perifollicular scales that "run away" from the hair forming a collar-like structure, which correspond to the scale crusts and aggregates of neutrophils on pathology (Figure 19.4); (3) folds of perifollicular epidermal hyperplasia in a starburst pattern, which corresponds to the follicular and interfollicular epidermal hyperplasia and the dermal fibrosis with loss of elastic fibers on pathology (Figure 19.5) and is more common in larger tufts; (4) other features: follicular pustules and elongated loop-like and coiled vessels in a concentric perifollicular arrangement (Figure 19.6), and white milky and ivory white areas devoid of follicular ostia in late disease (they correspond to the dermal fibrosis) (Figure 19.7).

MAIN HISTOLOGIC FEATURES

Typical FD Lesions

- Compounded follicular structures of 4, 5 or 6 follicles fused with their outer root sheaths at the level of the infundibulum (6-packs). We have suggested

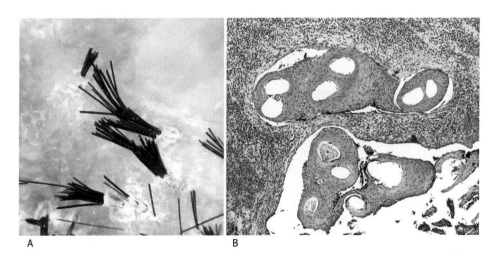

A   B

FIGURE 19.3 (A) On trichoscopy tufts of hairs (more than 6) come out of the same ostia and are surrounded by tubular white/yellow scale (×20). (B) Their histologic equivalent is the compound follicular structures formed by the fusion of the outer root sheaths of 6 or more follicles.

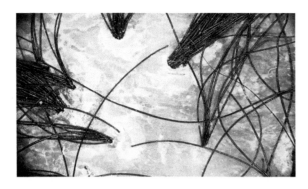

FIGURE 19.4 Prominent perifollicular white/yellow scales that "run away" from the tufts forming a collar-like structure; note the milky white interfollicular areas (×50). (Image courtesy of Giselle Martins, MD.)

the term "eyes" and "goggles" for the two packs (corresponding to the mini-tufts in lymphocytic cicatricial alopecia) and "monster goggles" for the multi-follicular packs in FD (Figures 19.3 and 19.8)
- Neutrophilic pustules in the follicular ostia (Figure 19.5)

- Loss of sebaceous glands (Figure 19.8)
- Dense perifollicular and interfollicular infiltrate of mixed cell origin (neutrophils, lymphocytes, histiocytes and plasma cells) predominantly at the upper follicular level (Figures 19.3, 19.5 and 19.8)
- Perifollicular concentric fibrosis (Figure 19.8)
- Fragmented hair shafts (Figure 19.9)
- Interfollicular acanthosis (vertical sections) (Figure 19.8)

FDLPPPS (See Also Chapter 13)

- *Compounded follicular structures* (e.g. follicular packs) of 2–5 follicles at the level of the upper isthmus and infundibulum, which differs from the common 6 and more packs in the typical FD presentation (Figure 19.10)
- *Atrophy of the follicular epithelium* (reduced thickness of the normally multilayered outer root sheath at the isthmus level to one/few layers) with perifollicular fibrosis and moderately dense or dense

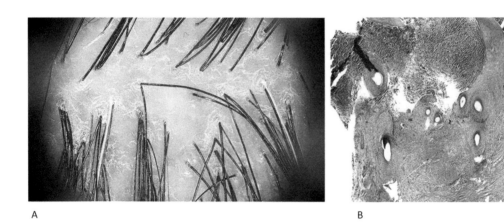

A   B

FIGURE 19.5   (A) A starburst sign surrounding the tufts of hairs (×40) corresponds to epidermal hyperplasia (black arrows) surrounding the compound follicular infundibula (B). Note the presence of dense mixed cell infiltrate, which corresponds to pustules and scale crusts, and the dermal fibrosis (yellow arrow).

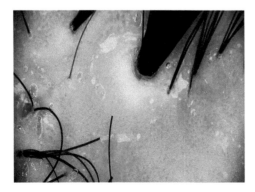

FIGURE 19.6   Concentric elongated perifollicular vessels in folliculitis decalvans(×60). (Image courtesy of Giselle Martins, MD.)

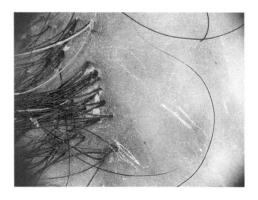

FIGURE 19.7   Milky white scarred areas devoid of follicular ostia (×40).

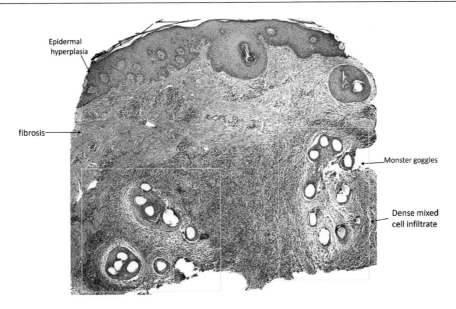

FIGURE 19.8 Classic histologic example of FD featuring "monster goggles" (6-or-more packs of hair follicles brought together by fusion of the outer root sheaths, ORS) at the infundibular level. Note the prominent atrophy of the ORS.

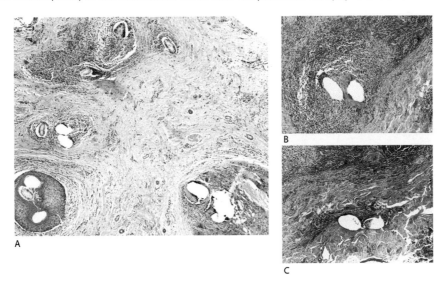

FIGURE 19.9 (A) Fragmented hair shafts with granulomatous infiltrate. Sometimes, the follicular epithelium is completely destroyed and only the holes marking the sites of the hair shafts remain in the dermis ("ghost goggles") (B, C).

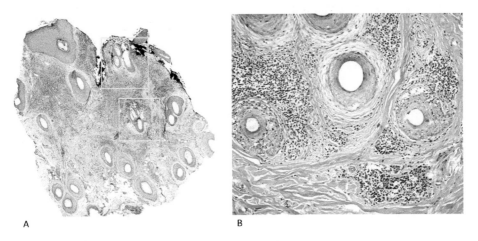

FIGURE 19.10 (A) FDLPPPS presents with smaller follicular packs (usually 2–5) as shown in this low power image. (B) The infiltrate is predominantly of plasma cells.

lichenoid and interstitial infiltrate of lymphocytes and plasma cells (Figure 19.11)

- *Plasma cells* are prominent, extending in aggregates in the deep dermis and in the subcutaneous fat (Figure 19.12)
- *Granulomas* (perifollicular granulomatous infiltrate around fragmented hair shafts)
- *Absent neutrophils*
- *Interfollicular acanthosis* (vertical sections) (Figure 19.10)
- *Follicular dropout and dermal fibrosis* (Figure 19.11)

PEARLS

- Trichoscopy with trichoscopy-guided scalp biopsies and bacterial cultures are the mainstay of the workup.
- Reporting the pathologic features with details on the type of inflammation (neutrophils in the typical cases and plasma cells in the FDLPPPS cases), presence of granulomas and interfollicular fibrosis is important to guide the management.

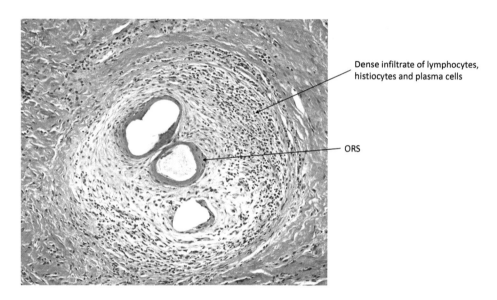

Dense infiltrate of lymphocytes, histiocytes and plasma cells

ORS

FIGURE 19.11   Atrophy of the follicular epithelium with almost complete consumption of the ORS. Note the perifollicular but also the dermal fibrosis.

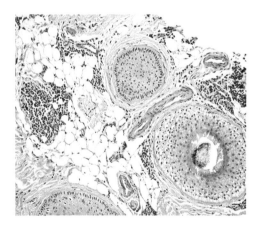

FIGURE 19.12   Collections of plasma cells in the subdermis.

FURTHER READING

Annessi G. Tufted folliculitis of the scalp: a distinctive clinicohistological variant of folliculitis decalvans. Br J Dermatol. 1998 May;138(5):799–805.

Egger A, Stojadinovic O, Miteva M. Folliculitis decalvans and lichen planopilaris phenotypic spectrum—A series of 7 new cases with focus on histopathology. Am J Dermatopathol. 2020 Mar;42(3):173–7.

Moreno-Arrones OM, Campo RD, Saceda-Corralo D, Jimenez-Cauhe J, Ponce-Alonso M, Serrano-Villar S, Jaén P, Paoli J, Vañó-Galván S. Folliculitis decalvans microbiological signature is specific for disease clinical phenotype. J Am Acad Dermatol. 2020 Oct 31:S0190-9622(20)32894-2.

Rudnicka, L, Oszewska M, Rakowska A, eds. *Atlas of Trichoscopy – Dermoscopy in Hair and Scalp Disease*. 1st ed. London: Springer-Verlag; 2012:319–29.

Uchiyama M, Harada K, Tobita R, Irisawa R, Tsuboi R. Histopathologic and dermoscopic features of 42 cases of folliculitis decalvans: a case series. J Am Acad Dermatol. 2020 Apr 6:S0190-9622(20)30515-6.

Yip L, Barrett TH, Harries MJ. Folliculitis decalvans and lichen planopilaris phenotypic spectrum: a case series of biphasic clinical presentation and theories on pathogenesis. Clin Exp Dermatol. 2020 Jan;45(1):63–72.

Dissecting Cellulitis of the Scalp

20

Contents

GENERAL CONCEPTS

Dissecting cellulitis of the scalp (DCS) (perifolliculitis capitis abscedens et suffodiens) is a neutrophilic cicatricial alopecia characterized by inflammatory cystic nodules, plaques and sinuses that progress to permanent scarring in localized patchy or extensive cerebriform pattern; it mostly affects the vertex and occipital scalp of African American men.

- Although DCS falls in the same category with folliculitis decalvans, i.e. neutrophilic cicatricial alopecia, it has a very distinct clinical presentation that starts with *follicular occlusion*. Follicular occlusion is the underlying mechanism in the pathogenesis of hidradenitis suppurativa, acne conglobata and pilonidal cysts, which may be associated with DCS (the association is referred to as the follicular occlusion triad/tetrad).
- The initial lesions are comedonal-like structures (follicular occlusion) that lead to dense inflammatory response in the shape of pustules, fluctuant boggy nodules and sterile abscesses with granulation tissue. The lesions can be patchy and simulate alopecia areata (Figure 20.1). If left untreated, the lesions eventually result in interconnecting (cerebriform) sinus tracts (epithelial structures surrounding the abscess in the dermis) with overlying permanent alopecia (Figure 20.2); but if successfully and timely treated, partial regrowth is possible (Figure 20.1).
- The pathogenesis is unclear but genetic (proven familial occurrences), hormonal (male sex and

localization on the vertex) and possibly environmental factors may play a role. Other culprits include neutrophils, especially via interleukin-1, microbiota may play an important role as alloantigens and lost immune tolerance to alloantigens in the hair follicle may lead to an inflammatory reaction.

- The lesions are sterile; however, secondary bacterial infection most commonly with coagulase-negative staphylococci may occur.
- Involvement of the lower portion of the hair follicles by the inflammation leads to premature shift into telogen (similar to alopecia areata), which results in increased shedding. The follicle is unable to start a new anagen phase and remains empty, accumulating sebum and keratin. Treatment can lead to regrowth at this early stage (Figure 20.1).
- On *trichoscopy,* there are (1) double-bordered 3D-yellow dots which correspond to the occluded follicular ostia with sebum and keratin, with or without centrally located black dots, which correspond to dystrophic hairs at the skin surface as a result of abrupt telogen shift (Figure 20.3); (2) some 3D yellow dots contain less well-defined black dots that are reminiscent of the hair powder sign in trichotillomania (see Chapter 12) as they correspond to pigmented casts from trichomalacia (Figure 20.4); (3) a yellow/violaceous structureless area that corresponds to the inflammation in the dermis (Figure 20.3); (4) cutaneous clefts containing hair shafts (usually 5–8 hairs) are noted in the later stage when fibrosis occurs. These are not hair tufts per se as they do no form

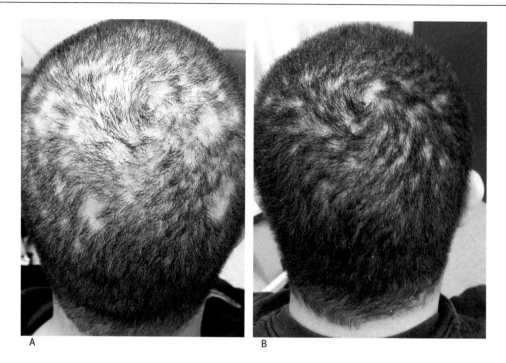

FIGURE 20.1   (A) Erythematous hairless patches at first visit and (B) significant regrowth after treatment.

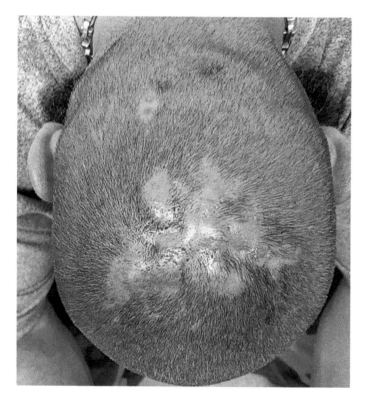

FIGURE 20.2   Boggy areas of scarring alopecia in DCS.

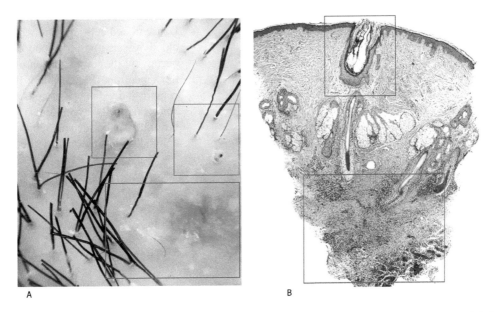

A   B

FIGURE 20.3   Double-bordered 3D yellow dots on trichoscopy (A, ×20) correspond on histology (B) to dilated follicular infundibula packed with sebum and keratin; the violaceous structureless area is due to dense diffuse dermal inflammation. Note also the black dots and broken hairs.

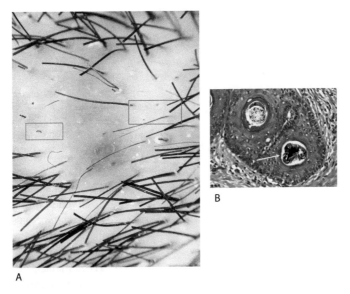

B

A

FIGURE 20.4   Another example of DCS showing the powder sign (less well-defined black dots) (A, ×20) that correspond on histology (B) to trichomalacia with pigmented casts in the follicular ostia.

from fused outer root sheaths at the infundibular level but these are individual hairs brought together in a pocket of fibrosis in the remodeled dermis. The clefts are analogical to to the bridging and circinate scars with hollows in hidradenitis suppurativa; and (5) linear scars overlying healed sinus tracts (Figure 20.5).

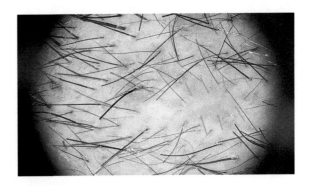

FIGURE 20.5   A linear scar overlying a healed sinus tract.

MAIN HISTOLOGIC FEATURES

- Trichoscopy-guided biopsy should be obtained from the 3D yellow dots and any area with black dots.
- A pustule is not an optimal site for a biopsy as the histologic yield may be lower due to non-specific mixed cell infiltrate.

- **Early disease**
  - Dense mixed cell infiltrate with edema, dilated blood vessels and red blood cell extravasation occupying the lower portion of the dermis and the subdermis (Figure 20.6); the infiltrate may contain individual giant cells or collections of epithelioid cells (granulomas) (Figure 20.7); the infiltrate can be seen also in the fibrous streamers and within the eccrine ducts (Figure 20.8)

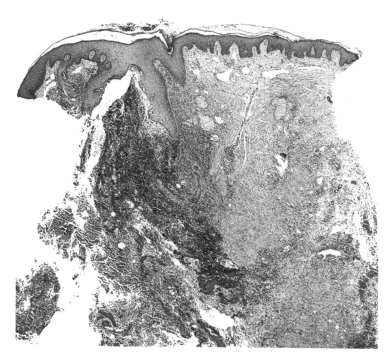

FIGURE 20.6 A ruptured infundibular cystic structure with significant superficial and deep abscess-like mixed cell infiltrate with dilated vessels and red blood cell extravasation.

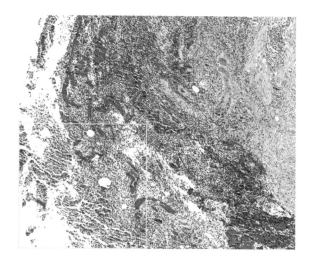

FIGURE 20.7 Epithelioid cell collections in the infiltrate.

The latter holds similarity with the apocrinitis observed in hidradenitis suppurativa
- Dilated infundibula plugged with keratin and sebum that correspond to the 3D yellow dots (Figure 20.3)
- Increased telogen count (Figure 20.9)
- Trichomalacia (fragmented hair shafts with pigmented casts in the follicular infundibula) (Figure 20.4)

- **Later disease**
  - Sebaceous glands can be partially or completely lost (Figure 20.10)
  - Follicular dropout
  - Chronic granulomatous infiltrate
  - Sinus tracts in the dermis (epithelial structures surrounding the abscess in the dermis form narrow opening or passageway extending from underneath the skin in any direction and results in dead space with potential for abscess formation) (Figures 20.10 and 20.11)
  - Fragmented hair shafts in the dermis and subdermis (Figure 20.12)
  - Dermal fibrosis (Figures 20.10 and 20.11)

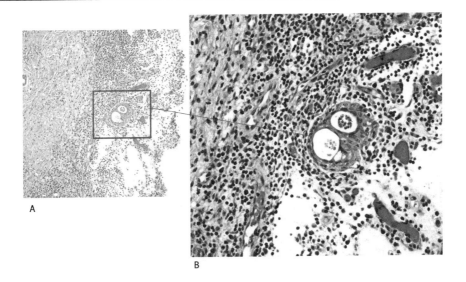

FIGURE 20.8 (A, B) Inflammation of the sweat ducts in DCS.

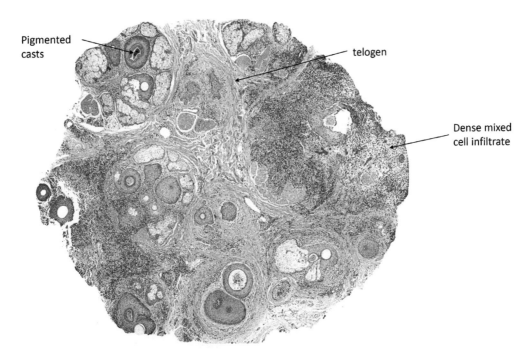

FIGURE 20.9 DCS on horizontal sections at the isthmus level.

PEARLS

- Early cases of DSC should be distinguished from alopecia areata by obtaining a biopsy as the clinical and trichoscopic features can be similar.
- DCS should be distinguished from inflammatory tinea capitis mimicking DCS, which may show similar clinical features; a complete workup with trichoscopy, histology and fungal culture should be performed at the same time as a single diagnostic test may fail to capture the diagnosis; a histologic clue in tinea capitis mimicking DCS is that the abscess-like dense inflammation extends from the follicular bulbs to the infundibular level (see Chapter 28).
- Always perform special stains for fungal infection in any biopsies ruling out DCS.
- In FD, there is a fusion of the outer root sheath of several follicles and the inflammatory infiltrate is rather folliculocentric with concentric perifollicular fibrosis; whereas in DCS, the inflammatory infiltrate is diffuse, moderately dense to dense in an abscess-like pattern, and there is mainly interfollicular dermal fibrosis, and only mild perifollicular fibrosis can be seen focally (Figure 20.9).

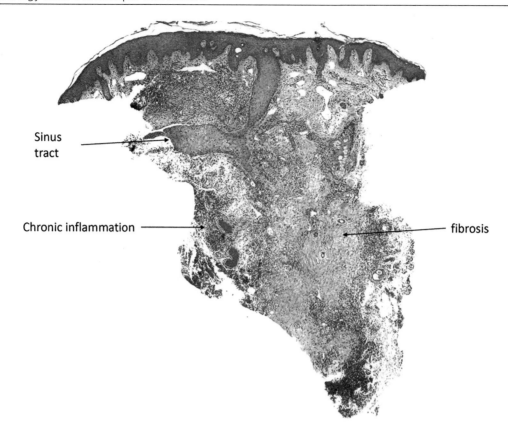

FIGURE 20.10   Loss of sebaceous glands, dermal fibrosis and sinus tracts in a later-stage DCS.

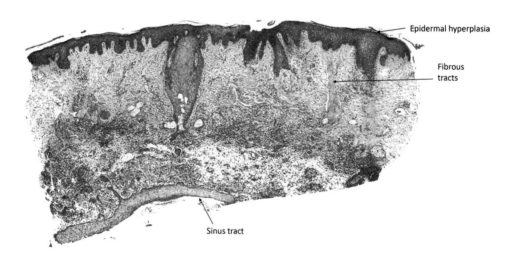

FIGURE 20.11   Another example of later-stage DCS with active inflammation and sinus tracts.

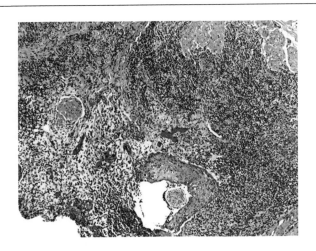

FIGURE 20.12 Follicular rupture with naked hair shaft among the dense inflammatory infiltrate.

Kong HH, Segre JA. Skin microbiome: looking back to move forward. J Invest Dermatol. 2012 Mar;132(3 Pt 2):933–9.

Lacarrubba F, Musumeci ML, Nasca MR, Verzì AE, Fiorentini F, Micali G. Double-ended pseudocomedones in hidradenitis suppurativa: clinical, dermoscopic, and histopatho-logical correlation. Acta Derm Venereol. 2017 Jun 9;97(6):763–764.

LaSenna CE, Miteva M, Tosti A. Pitfalls in the diagnosis of kerion. J Eur Acad Dermatol Venereol. 2016 Mar;30(3):515–7. doi: 10.1111/jdv.12912

Melo, D, Lemes, L, Pirmez, R, Duque-Estrada, B. Trichoscopic stages of dissecting cellulitis: a potential complementary tool to clinical assessment. Anais Brasileiros de Dermatologia. 2020;95(4):514–7.

Rudnicka, L, Oszewska M, Rakowska A, eds. *Atlas of Trichoscopy – Dermoscopy in Hair and Scalp Disease.* 1st ed. London: Springer-Verlag; 2012:331–7.

Saceda-Corralo D et al. Dissecting cellulitis of the scalp. In Miteva M, ed. *Alopecia.* 1st ed. Elsevier, 2018: 167–72.

Tosti A, Torres F, Miteva M. Dermoscopy of early dissecting cellulitis of the scalp simulates alopecia areata. Actas Dermosifiliogr. 2013 Jan;104(1):92–3.

FURTHER READING

Badaoui A, Reygagne P, Cavelier-Balloy B, Pinquier L, Deschamps L, Crickx B, Descamps V. Dissecting cellulitis of the scalp: a retrospective study of 51 patients and review of literature. Br J Dermatol. 2016 Feb;174(2):421–3.

Erosive Pustular Dermatosis of the Scalp

21

Contents

GENERAL CONCEPTS

Erosive pustular dermatosis of the scalp (EPDS) is a rare condition characterized by sterile pustules and erosions with superficial crusts that typically develop in longstanding atrophic sun-damaged skin of elderly patients; it may lead to scarring alopecia in cases with extensive involvement.

- Other names include "Chronic atrophic dermatosis of the scalp and extremities" since involvement of the leg as a chronic vegetating pyoderma has been reported in patients with chronic venous insufficiency.
- Atrophic (actinic) skin seems to be a prerequisite for the development of EPDS.
- Trauma and tissue damage seem to play the triggering role: preceding herpes zoster, iatrogenic injury caused by cryotherapy, carbon dioxide laser, topical chemotherapy for field cancerization, excisional surgery, imiquimod, tretinoin, grafting after surgery, x-ray radiation, and topical photodynamic therapy have been reported in association.
- The most common location is the vertex and the clinical presentation ranges from a few erosive, scaly lesions to crusted and hemorrhagic plaques, mimicking pustular pyoderma gangrenosum (Figures 21.1 and 21.2).
- The lesions usually have a linear distribution.
- There is variant with hypergranulation overlying the erosions.
- The pathogenies remains unclear. Factors such as loss of normal epidermal barrier and tissue damage may induce a reaction of immune dysregulation in the hair follicle and therefore some consider EPDS a neutrophilic superficial folliculitis, part of the spectrum of pathergic neutrophilic dermatoses such as pyoderma gangrenosum.
- On *trichoscopy, there are non-specific features* but distinctions between active and chronic cases can be made according to Starace et al.
  - **Active disease:** The most characteristic finding is the anagen bulb visible thought the atrophic skin; other features include yellow-hemorrhagic crusts, pili torti, dystrophic hairs and mini-tufts of 2–4 hairs emerging together from the same ostium (Figures 21.3 and 21.4)
  - **Chronic disease:** Significantly atrophic skin with visible anagen bulbs, lack of follicular ostia (Figure 21.5), yellow exudate
  - **Vessels in EPDS:** Enlarged and polymorphous vessels have been described, particularly in the hypergranulation variant

MAIN HISTOLOGIC FEATURES

The histologic features are non-specific.

- **Active and early disease**
  - The inflammation is centered in the mid and upper follicle (infundibulo-folliculitis), and the lower follicular levels are unaffected (Figure 21.6)
  - Normal follicular density with increased telogen count

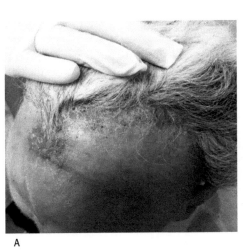
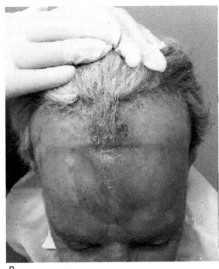

FIGURE 21.1 (A, B) EPDS in a patient with sun-damaged skin which developed after partial thickness skin graft for squamous cell carcinoma. (Courtesy of Giselle Martins, MD.)

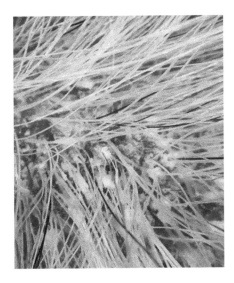

FIGURE 21.2 Diffuse erythema and yellow scale crusts on clinical exam. (Courtesy of Giselle Martins, MD.)

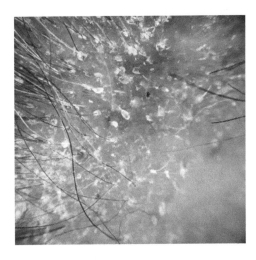

FIGURE 21.3 Yellow crusts, diffuse erythema in active disease (×20). (Courtesy of Giselle Martins, MD.)

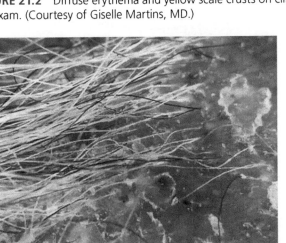

FIGURE 21.4 Pustules and yellow exudate (×20). (Courtesy of Giselle Martins, MD.)

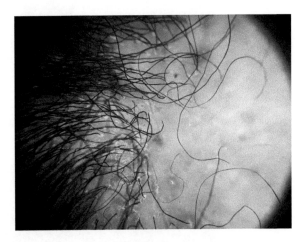

FIGURE 21.5 Loss of follicular ostia, milky white areas of scarring, broken hairs, pili torti-like hairs (×20). (Courtesy of Giselle Martins, MD.)

– Edema and polymorphous dermal inflammatory infiltrate of neutrophils, lymphocytes, plasma cells, rare eosinophils and foreign body giant cells in the dermis (Figures 21.6–21.9)
– Spongiform pustules on the top of some follicular orifices or within the epidermis have been described (Figure 21.8)

– The epidermis may show psoriasiform acanthosis (Figure 21.8)

• **Chronic disease**
– Laminated compact orthokeratosis and epidermal atrophy
– Follicular dropout
– Absence of sebaceous glands
– Diffuse and severe fibrosis in the dermis

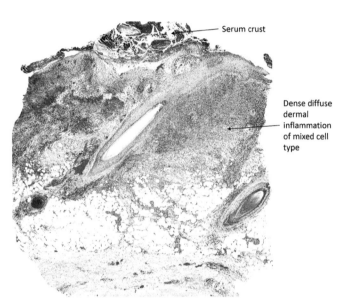

FIGURE 21.6   EPDS shows edema and dense polymorphous infiltrate most pronounced in the upper and mid-dermis.

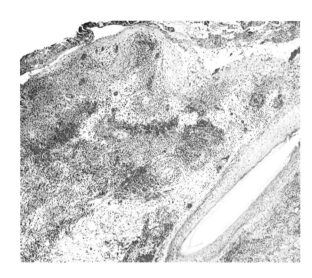

FIGURE 21.7   The infiltrate contains lymphocytes, histiocytes, plasma cells, neutrophils and eosinophils, and there is pronounced red blood cell extravasation.

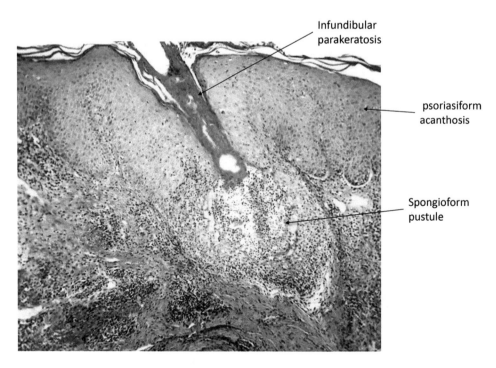

FIGURE 21.8   Infundibulocentric spongiform pustule (arrow). (Courtesy of Ana Leticia Boff, MD.)

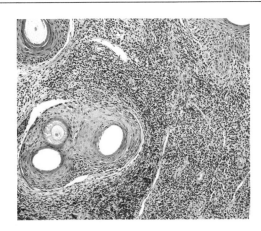

FIGURE 21.9 Biopsy, from the same patient as in Figures 21.6 and 21.7, on horizontal sections shows a compound follicular structure with dense upper dermal mixed cell infiltrate. There is only mild perifollicular fibrosis, which could also be absent.

- Compared with dissecting cellulitis of the scalp (DCS) and folliculitis decalvans (FD), the inflammatory infiltrate is more superficial and centered at the isthmo-infundibular level (vs. the lower level in DCS), and there is none or only slight perifollicular fibrosis (vs. FD).
- Fungal stains need to be performed for completeness in order to exclude an inflammatory tinea capitis.

FURTHER READING

Laffitte E, Kaya G, Piguet V, Saurat J. Erosive pustular dermatosis of the scalp: treatment with topical tacrolimus. Arch Dermatol. 2003;139(6):712–714.

Semkova K, Tchernev G, Wollina U. Erosive pustular dermatosis (chronic atrophic dermatosis of the scalp and extremities). Clin Cosmet Investig Dermatol. 2013;6:177–182.

Starace M, Alessandrini A, Baraldi C, Piraccini BM. Erosive pustular dermatosis of the scalp: challenges and solutions. Clin Cosmet Investig Dermatol. 2019;12:691–698.

Starace M, Loi C, Bruni F, et al. Erosive pustular dermatosis of the scalp: clinical, trichoscopic, and histopathologic features of 20 cases. J Am Acad Dermatol. 2017;76(6):1109–1114.e2.

Starace M, Patrizi A, Piraccini BM. Visualisation of hair bulbs through the scalp: a trichoscopic feature of erosive pustular dermatosis of the scalp. Int J Trichol. 2016.

Tomasini, Carlo et al. Erosive pustular dermatosis of the scalp: a neutrophilic folliculitis within the spectrum of neutrophilic dermatoses; J Am Acad Dermatol. 2018;81(2):527–533.

PEARLS

- Linear crusted erosions on sun-damaged atrophic skin that has suffered some chemical or mechanical trauma point to EPDS; however, the clinical, trichoscopic and histologic features are non-specific and EPDS remains a diagnosis of exclusion.
- Long-term follow-up for the development of cutaneous malignancy is recommended.

Acne/Folliculitis Keloidalis

22

Contents

GENERAL CONCEPTS

Acne keloidalis/acne kleoidalis nuchae (AKN), also known as folliculitis keloidalis, is a primary neutrophilic cicatricial alopecia that mostly occurs in men of African, African American and Afro-Caribbean origin with coarse curly hair, and is characterized by chronic follicular papules mainly on the occipital scalp and neck that evolve into keloid-like scars and permanent alopecia.

- The name "keloidalis" is a misnomer as the lesions do not show keloidal features on histology and the patients do not have tendency to develop keloids in other parts of the body.
- The onset after puberty and the exclusive predilection for the male sex suggest a hormonal component in the pathogenesis.
- It is believed that chronic local mechanical irritation to the nuchal and the occipital area, by frequent shaving, picking or friction to hair that is kinky, leads to follicular irritation, exposure to follicular alloantigens that evoke an immune response with inflammation, follicular destruction and transepidermal elimination of the hair shafts in the dermis. This leads to further chronic inflammation with granulomas. The reparative attempts in predisposed individuals result in abnormal hypertrophic scarring and permanent alopecia.
- Metabolic syndrome (present in 61% of the patients as per a recent study) and chronic infection (*Demodex, Staphylococcus, Malassezia*) may play a secondary role in the pathogenesis.

- **Early lesions:** Flesh-colored or erythematous papules, with pustules on the occipital scalp and the posterior part of the neck that may extend into the vertex (Figure 22.1). The lesions are accompanied by itch or pain.
- **Late lesions:** Sclerotic plaques, nodules and keloidal masses with sinus tracts, and devoid of hairs (cicatricial alopecia) (Figure 22.2).
- Androgenetic alopecia, central centrifugal cicatricial alopecia and folliculitis decalvans have been reported in association with AKN.

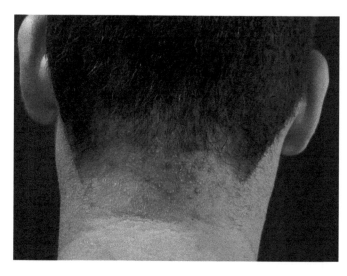

FIGURE 22.1 Erythematous papules, with pustules on the occipital scalp. (Courtesy of Giselle Martins, MD; reprinted with permission from Katoulis A, Ioannides D, Rigopoulos D, eds., *Hair Disorders: Diagnosis and Management*, CRC Press: Boca Raton and Abingdon, forthcoming 2021.)

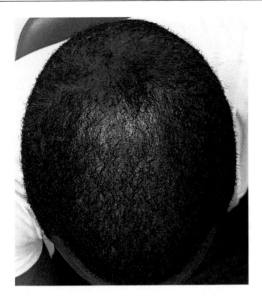

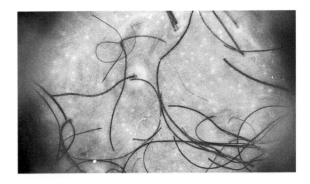

FIGURE 22.5 These late lesions show white folliculocentric papules and irregular pigmented network (×20). (Reprinted with permission from Katoulis A, Ioannides D, Rigopoulos D, eds., *Hair Disorders: Diagnosis and Management*, CRC Press: Boca Raton and Abingdon, forthcoming 2021.)

FIGURE 22.2 Folliculitis keloidalis resulting in patchy hairless cicatricial alopecia on the vertex.

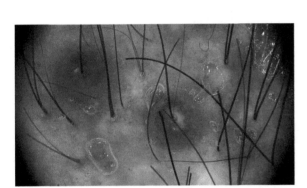

FIGURE 22.3 Early AKN: folliculocentric papules with a red rim (×40). (Courtesy of Giselle Martins, MD; reprinted with permission from Katoulis A, Ioannides D, Rigopoulos D, eds., *Hair Disorders: Diagnosis and Management*, CRC Press: Boca Raton and Abingdon, forthcoming 2021.)

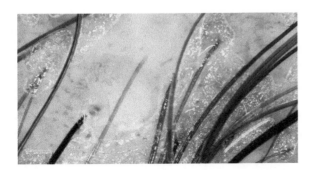

FIGURE 22.4 Folliculocentric papules with crown vessels (×60). (Courtesy to Giselle Martins, MD.)

- On *trichoscopy* the features depend on the stage:
  - **Early stage** shows folliculocentric pink papules and pustules with a red rim and white streaks (Figure 22.3) and crown vessels (Figure 22.4), which correspond to chronic inflammatory infiltrate and perifollicular fibrosis; broken hairs and peripilar casts ensue from the follicular destruction.
  - **Later stage** shows white follicular papules, white patches at the site of loss of follicular openings and irregular pinpoint white dots (Figure 22.5). Intact hair follicles at the margins may exhibit tufting.

MAIN HISTOLOGIC FEATURES

In individual small follicular scars and symptomatic papules, punch biopsies that extend to the fat can be done with diagnostic but also with a treatment purpose, as they can excise the entire affected hair follicle; silk sutures could be used as they cause less inflammation.

- **Early lesions**
  - Dilated follicular canals and fragmented hair shafts
  - Dense infiltrate of neutrophils, lymphocytes and many plasma cells are distributed around the isthmus and the lower infundibulum of the hair follicle
  - Sebaceous glands are absent
  - *Demodex* and *Malassezia* are detected within the sebaceous ducts in some patients

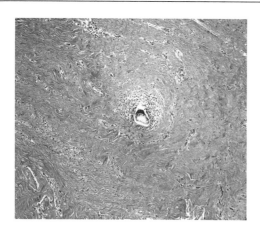

FIGURE 22.6 Fragmented hair shafts from ruptured follicles are surrounded by chronic inflammation and dense fibrosis. (Reprinted with permission from Katoulis A, Ioannides D, Rigopoulos D, eds., *Hair Disorders: Diagnosis and Management*, CRC Press: Boca Raton and Abingdon, forthcoming 2021.)

- **Late lesions**
  - Chronic granulomatous inflammation
  - Follicular dropout
  - Fragmented hair shafts (Figure 22.6)
  - Dense dermal fibrosis without keloidal features (i.e., absence of whorled masses of hyalinized glassy collagen) (Figure 22.7)

PEARLS

- Vertical sections are more appropriate for the diagnosis.

FURTHER READING

Herzberg AJ, Dinehart SM, Kerns BJ, Pollack SV. Acne keloidalis. Transverse microscopy, immunohistochemistry, and electron microscopy. Am J Dermatopathol. Apr 1990;12(2):109–121.

Miteva M, Sabiq S, Acne keloidalis nuchae, in Katoulis A, Ioannides D, Rigopoulos D, eds., *Hair Disorders: Diagnosis and Management*, CRC Press: Boca Raton and Abingdon, forthcoming 2021.

Na K, Oh SH, Kim SK. Acne keloidalis nuchae in Asian: A single institutional experience. PloS One. 2017;12(12):e0189790.

Ocampo-Garza J, Tosti A. Trichoscopy of Dark Scalp. Skin Appendage Disorders. Nov 2018;5(1):1–8.

Shapero J, Shapero H. Acne keloidalis nuchae is scar and keloid formation secondary to mechanically induced folliculitis. Journal of Cutaneous Medicine and Surgery. Jul–Aug 2011;15(4):238–240.

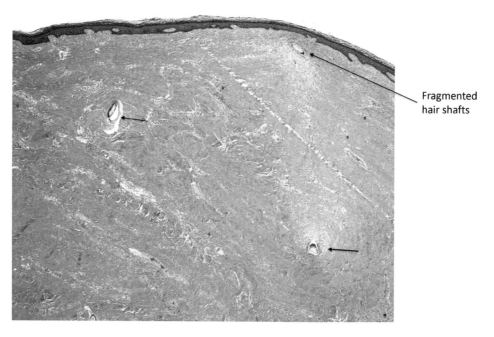

Fragmented hair shafts

FIGURE 22.7 Dense thick collagen effaces the normal dermal architecture. Note the absence of keloidal (glassy and whorled) collagen bundles. (Reprinted with permission from Katoulis A, Ioannides D, Rigopoulos D, eds., *Hair Disorders: Diagnosis and Management*, CRC Press: Boca Raton and Abingdon, forthcoming 2021.)

Scalp Psoriasis

23

Contents

Psoriasis is a common dermatological condition that involves the scalp in up to 80% of the cases and it can be the only clinical manifestation of the disease in about 30%. It presents as erythematous plaques of various thicknesses that are well circumscribed and covered by white/silver scales. Most common predilection sites are the hairline, including the retroauricular area; but any part of the scalp can be affected (Figure 23.1).

GENERAL CONCEPTS

- Three different types of alopecia can occur in scalp psoriasis: (1) *patchy or diffuse alopecia* in the affected by psoriasis skin; (2) *telogen effluvium* – it usually commences with the initiation of successful

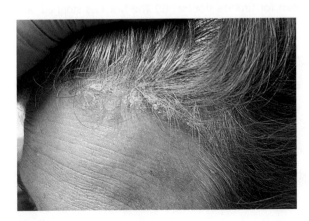

FIGURE 23.1 Classic example of psoriatic plaques involving the hairline.

local therapy that results in successful detachment of the thick scales and the telogen hairs entrapped in them; and very rarely (3) *scarring alopecia*.

- Paradoxically, an increased density of hair in psoriatic plaques has also been reported and it is believed that monocytes and macrophages could have a key role in the cascade of events leading to anagen switch-on by upregulation of the Wnt/β-catenin pathway.

- Most patients experience the regrowth of hair with a successful treatment, which is likely explained by the fact that psoriasis is a disease of the inter-follicular skin and the lower portion of the hair follicle is usually spared without significant inflammation (according to a comparative analysis by Ruano et al. on lesional and non-lesional samples from patients with untreated moderate to severe psoriasis and significant scalp involvement as well as control subjects without psoriasis).

- Scalp psoriasis has a Th1/Th17 cytokine activation profile, similar to skin psoriasis.

- The inflammation in psoriatic alopecia is centered mainly at the infundibulum and therefore it is unlikely that scarring alopecia in psoriasis is primary in nature; it most likely occurs in prolonged cases with superinfection. The constant lack of sebum in scalp psoriasis decreases the antimicrobial resistance in the affected skin.

- Alopecia areata has been reported in association with psoriasis; however, the resolution of alopecia areata in the psoriatic scalp has been described as well (referred to as the Renbök phenomenon).

- An overlap pattern with concomitant clinical features for psoriasis and seborrheic dermatitis has been referred to as sebopsoriasis, and whereas it is a convenient clinical term for the daily practice, it lacks clear diagnostic criteria, including on histology.

- **Psoriatic alopecia areata-like reaction to TNF-alpha inhibitors:** This is considered a paradoxical reaction as these drugs are utilized to treat psoriasis; it usually occurs in patients without prior personal or family history of psoriasis who receive infliximab or adalimumab for Crohn's disease, ankylosing spondylitis or rheumatoid arthritis.
  - The most common clinical presentation is psoriasiform plaques with or without patchy or diffuse alopecia (Figure 23.2).
  - On *trichoscopy*, apart from the features for psoriasis, black dots, broken hairs and circle hairs can be noticed as in alopecia areata (Figure 23.3).
  - Common association is palmo-plantar pustular psoriasis.
  - Resolution with topical therapy is possible in milder cases but more severe cases require switching to a biologic alternative from a different category (Figure 23.2).

- **Psoriatic alopecia-like reaction due to IL17-inhibitors** with a similar clinical and histologic

presentation has been reported with ixekizumab but can occur also with secukinumab (personal observation) (Figures 23.4 and 23.5).

On *trichosopy,* the vascular pattern is the most characteristic finding.

On *dry trichoscopy* and low magnification, only thick diffuse interfollicular white scaling overlying erythematous background can be appreciated (Figure 23.6). If the scale is hydrated, red dots and globules are found (Figure 23.7). Using *a higher magnification (>50) on videodermoscopy* identifies the red globules to be glomerular/coiled vessels, which are organized in clusters or in string-like linear pattern (the latter being similar to the pattern in clear cell acanthoma) (Figure 23.8). In small individual lesions, especially on sun-damaged skin, Bowen's disease must be excluded by histology. Other type of vessels such as loops, lace-like or linear coiled vessels can be seen arranged in a pattern in the same plaque (Figure 23.9).

MAIN HISTOLOGIC FEATURES

Classic plaques are rarely biopsied. Both vertical and horizontal sections can be useful for the diagnosis. If only one biopsy

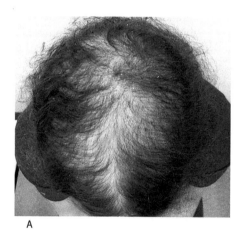
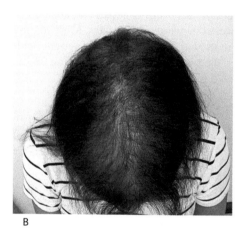

A   B

FIGURE 23.2   (A) Diffuse psoriatic alopecia in a patient on adalimumab for Crohn's disease. (B) The hair loss stopped and hair regrowth occurred 2 months after discontinuing the drug.

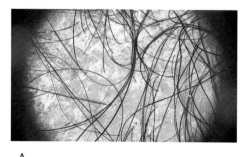
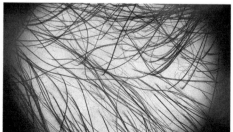

A   B

FIGURE 23.3   Same case (as in Figure 23.2) showing thick interfollicular scale on dry trichoscopy (A, ×20) and short regrowing hairs and circle hairs with improvement (B, ×20).

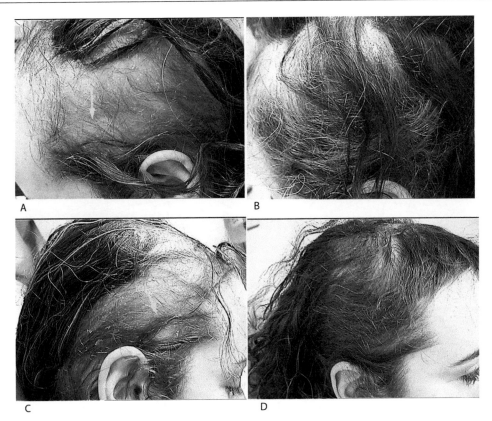

FIGURE 23.4 (A, C) Diffuse and patchy alopecia-areata like psoriatic alopecia in a patient on secukinumab for psoriasis. (B, D) Improvement after discontinuing the drug and using topical steroids and minoxidil.

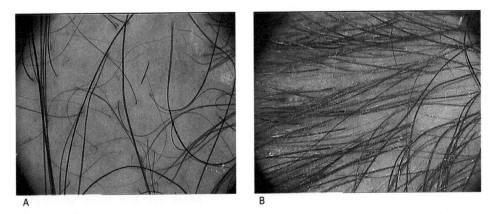

FIGURE 23.5 Same case (as in Figure 23.4) showing (A) dystrophic hairs on trichoscopy and (B) upright regrowing hairs with improvement.

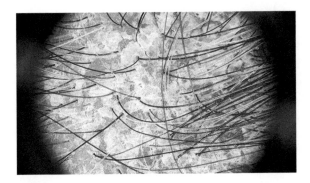

FIGURE 23.6 Thick diffuse interfollicular white-silver scaling overlying erythematous background (×20).

specimen is available and the ruling out diagnosis is psoriasis, vertical sectioning should be preferred.

- Psoriasiform acanthosis (uniform epidermal hyperplasia) with suprapapillary thinning and hypogranulosis
- Irregular epidermal hyperplasia is seen in many specimens especially if lesions have been treated (Figures 23.10, 23.11 and 23.12)
- Confluent parakeratosis with neutrophils in the stratum corneum (Figure 23.10)
- Spongiosis and necrotic keratinocytes (two features that are not encountered in psoriasis on glabrous skin) (Figure 23.10)

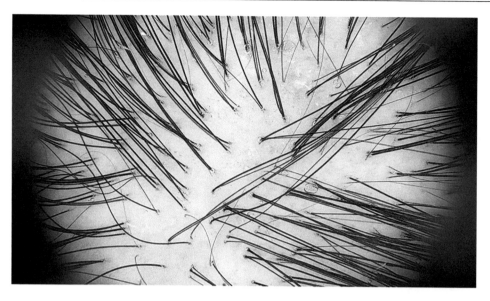

FIGURE 23.7   After hydrating the scale with an immersion fluid red dots and globules are noted (×20).

- Prominent tortuous vessels in the dermal papillae (Figure 23.11)
- An increased telogen count (Figures 23.11 and 23.12)
- Atrophy or absence of the sebaceous glands (Figures 23.11, 23.14 and 23.15)
- On *horizontal sections*, the atrophic sebaceous glands are present as thin epithelial strands

(mantle-like structures) or as small sprouts of hypoplastic sebaceous lobules (Figures 23.13, 23.14 and 23.15). The follicular epithelium shows infundibular acanthosis, which in some cases may resemble the gear wheel-like structures in lichen simplex chronicus (Figure 23.16). The telogen increase is easier appreciated on horizontal sections (Figure 23.17)
- In psoriatic alopecia due to TNF-alpha inhibitors, the features are similar to those in scalp psoriasis with prominent increased telogen count and numerous eosinophils and plasma cells in the inflammatory infiltrate that extends into the fat and can be found also in the fibrous streamers

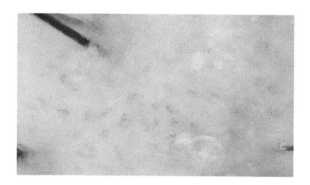

FIGURE 23.8   Coiled vessels on higher magnification (×70).

PEARLS

- In psoriasis, the architecture of the lower portion of the hair follicles is largely preserved without a significant immune infiltrate, likely explaining why

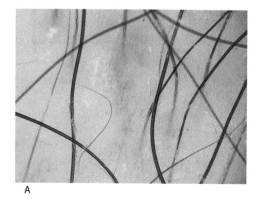

A

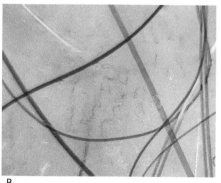

B

FIGURE 23.9   Lace-like vessels in clusters on higher magnification (×70).

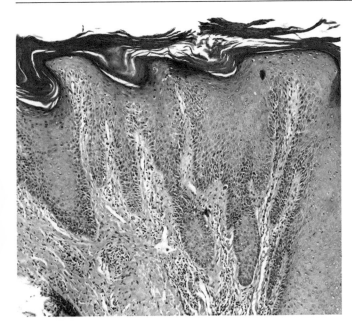

FIGURE 23.10 Irregular hyperplasia (irregular length of the elongated rete ridges) with confluent parakeratosis. There is also mild spongiosis.

- alopecia is rare and potential for hair regrowth is intact.
- In patients with scalp psoriasis and androgenetic alopecia, using an oral treatment (for instance, oral vs. topical minoxidil) avoids the friction and telogen shedding ensuing from the topical application and therefore could be a better therapeutic strategy.
- Patients with connective tissue disease, particularly dermatomyositis, lupus erythematous and mixed connective tissue disease may present with psoriasiform scalp dermatitis. In such cases, the presence

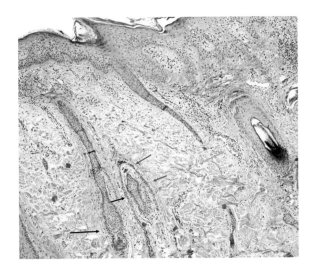

FIGURE 23.11 Irregular epidermal hyperplasia. Note the superficial perivascular lymphocytic infiltrate and increased telogen count (black arrows) with atrophic sebaceous glands (red arrows). Note the tortuous dilated vessels (green arrows).

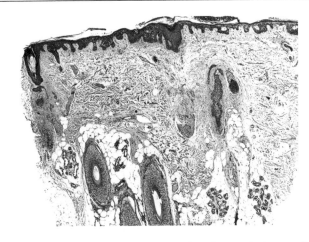

FIGURE 23.12 Another example of scalp psoriasis revealing irregular epidermal hyperplasia, atrophic sebaceous glands and telogen follicles.

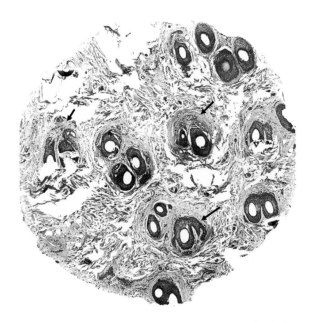

FIGURE 23.13 Horizontal sections at the isthmus level show the striking absence of sebaceous glands, which remain as mantle-like epithelial structures projecting from the follicular epithelium (arrows).

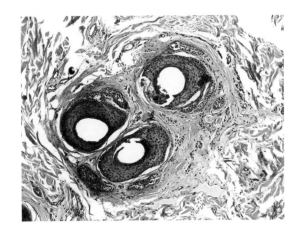

FIGURE 23.14 Atrophy of the sebaceous glands in psoriasis.

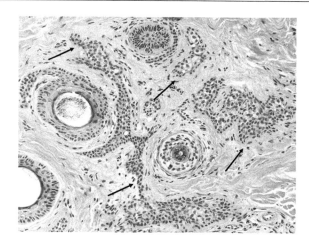

FIGURE 23.15 Prominent atrophy of the sebaceous glands (arrows).

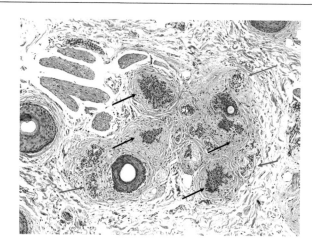

FIGURE 23.17 Increased telogen count (black arrows) and hypoplastic sebaceous glands at the isthmus level (red arrows).

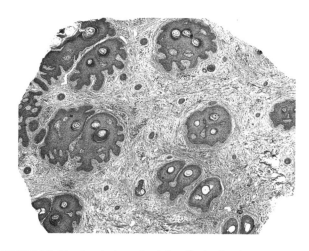

FIGURE 23.16 Psoriasis at the infundibular level. Note the pronounced acanthosis projecting from the follicular epithelium in a gear wheel-like pattern.

of giant enlarged capillaries on trichoscopy can be a distinguishing feature. Searching for other distinctive clinical features outside the scalp and obtaining a scalp biopsy provides further help with the diagnosis (Figure 23.18).

- Scalp biopsies with atrophy or absence of the sebaceous glands should not be immediately diagnosed as scarring alopecia. Atrophy of the sebaceous glands is a physiologic feature of prepuberty, menopause/adrenopause, scalp psoriasis and lichen simplex chronicus.

FURTHER READING

Doyle LA, Sperling LC, Baksh S, Lackey J, Thomas B, Vleugels RA, Qureshi AA, Velazquez EF. Psoriatic alopecia/alopecia areata-like reactions secondary to anti-tumor necrosis factor-α therapy: a novel cause of noncicatricial alopecia. Am J Dermatopathol. 2011 Apr;33(2):161–6.

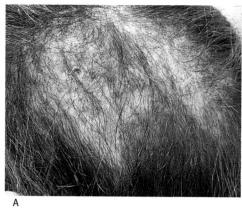

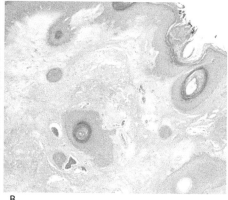

A   B

FIGURE 23.18 (A) Psoriasiform dermatitis in a patient with mixed connective tissue disease. (B) On biopsy, there is hyperkeratosis, follicular plugging, thickened basement membrane and mucin in the dermis, which confirm the diagnosis.

El-Shabrawi-Caelen L. Scalp psoriasis. In Miteva M, ed. *Alopecia.*, 1st ed. Elsevier, 2018:229–34.

George SM, Taylor MR, Farrant PB. Psoriatic alopecia. Clinic Exp Dermatol. 2015 40(7):717–21.

Hafeez F, Miteva M. SnapshotDx quiz: September 2016. J Invest Dermatol. 2016 Sep;136(9):e95.

Ruano J, Suárez-Fariñas M, Shemer A, Oliva M, Guttman-Yassky E, Krueger JG. Molecular and cellular profiling of scalp psoriasis reveals differences and similarities compared to skin psoriasis. PLoS One 5;11(2):e0148450.

Rudnicka, L, Oszewska M, Rakowska A, eds. *Atlas of Trichoscopy – Dermoscopy in Hair and Scalp Disease.* 1st ed. London: Springer-Verlag; 2012:379–89.

Sawan S, Descamps V. Scalp psoriasis: a paradigm of "switch-on" mechanism to anagen hair growth? Arch Dermatol. 2008;144(8):1064–6.

Tan TL, Taglia L, Yazdan P. Drug-induced psoriasiform alopecia associated with interleukin-17 inhibitor therapy. J Cutan Pathol. 2021 Jan 2.

Werner B, Brenner FM, Böer A. Histopathologic study of scalp psoriasis: peculiar features including sebaceous gland atrophy. Am J Dermatopathol. 2008;30(2):93–100.

Seborrheic Dermatitis

24

Contents

Seborrehic dermatitis (SD) is a common chronic inflammatory skin condition of the scalp and other regions rich in sebaceous glands (central face and anterior chest) that presents with erythematous thin patches or scaly plaques covered by yellowish moist greasy scales.

GENERAL CONCEPTS

- SD has a relapsing course and is more prevalent in patients with immunodifficencies, neurologic conditions and higher body fat content.
- Clinical variants include pityriasis capitis (dandruff), crusta lactea (cradle cap) in inflants, seborrhea petaloides or annular seborrheic dermatitis in patients of darker skin type, and tinea amiantacea (Figure 24.1).

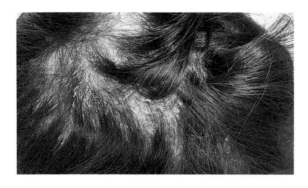

FIGURE 24.1 Tinea amiantacea (asbestos-like tinea) in a patient with history of seborrheic dermatitis presents with thick heavy yellow scales.

- Some cases with retroauricular involvement are indistinguishable from psoriasis and are often referred to as sebopsoriasis.
- The pathogenesis has not been fully elucidated, but *Malassezia* species have been considered a criticial factor due to their lipase activity leading to release of inflammatory free fatty acids and their ability to activate the alternative complement pathway. However, intrinsic host factors, such as changes in the amount or composition of sebum and/or defective epidermal barrier, rather than abnormal host response to *Malassezia* spp., are currently the favored pathogenic factors.
- On *trichoscopy,* SD is characterized by (1) yellow greasy interfollicular scaling that is appreciated only on dry trichoscopy (Figure 24.2). If the scale is hydrated, the yellow color remains as a background (Figure 24.3). In tinea amiantacea, there is thick white-yellow compact keratotic material that extends onto the hairs and binds together their proximal portions (asbestos-like scale) (Figure 24.4). (2) The most characteristic is the vascular pattern that includes multiple thin arborizing vessels in irregular distribution and atypical red vessels but absence of red dots and globules (Figures 24.3, 24.5 and 24.6).

MAIN HISTOLOGIC FEATURES

Classic scalp SD is rarely biopsied. The histologic findings depend on the age of the lesion biopsied.

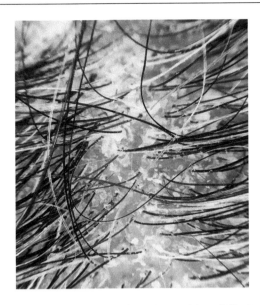

FIGURE 24.2 Yellow greasy follicular and interfollicular scales in SD (×20).

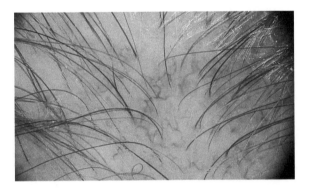

FIGURE 24.3 After hydrating the scale, a yellow background remains in seborrheic dermatitis; note the irregularly distributed thin arborizing vessels (×50). (Courtesy of Giselle Martins, MD.)

- **Acute lesions**
  - A mild spongiosis with overlying scale crust that is often centered over a follicle in a shoulder-like pattern (Figures 24.7 and 24.8).
  - The papillary dermis may be edematous (Figure 24.9).
  - Dilated blood vessels in the superficial vascular plexus (Figure 24.9)
  - A mild superficial perivascular infiltrate of lymphocytes, histiocytes and occasional neutrophils (Figures 24.7 and 24.9). The infiltrate can be seen also around the follicular infundibula with mild fibroplasia (Figure 24.10).
  - The sebaceous ducts are dilated and the sebaceous glands are hypetrophic (Figure 24.11).
  - Yeast forms of *Malassezia* spp. can be detected in the stratum corneum and highlighted by the fungal stains (Figure 24.12).

- **Subacute lesions**
  - Psoraisiform hyperplasia and minimal spongiosis
  - A mild perifollicular fibroplasia is seen in some cases and should not be interpreted as a feature of scarring alopecia.

PEARLS

- Thin arborizing vessels on dermoscopy are normal finding in the occipital scalp (particularly in men).
- If seborrheic dermatitis is the only ruling out diagnosis, vertical sections should be preferred for the diagnosis. If the ruling out diagnosis is for instance diffuse non-scarring alopecia with seborrheic dermatitis, then horizontal sections are preferred as they allow for assessment of the

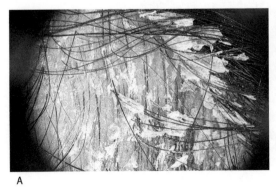
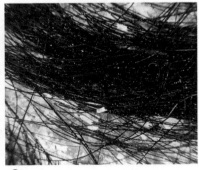

FIGURE 24.4 (A) Tinea amiantacea shows thick white-yellow compact keratotic material that extend onto the hairs and bind together their proximal portions. (B) The scales can be seen also extending along some hair shafts.

follicular architecture, and for follicular counts and ratios.

- In ambiguous cases of psoriasis vs. seborrheic dermatitis, the intact/hyperplastic sebaceous glands point to seborrheic dermatitis as psoriasis is characterized by atrophy of the sebaceous glands.

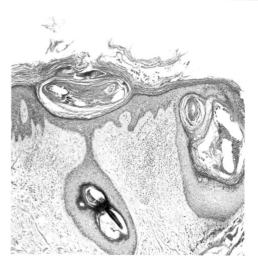

FIGURE 24.7 Dilated infundibula covered with parakeratosis. Note the mild dermal inflammatory infiltrate and the irregular acanthosis.

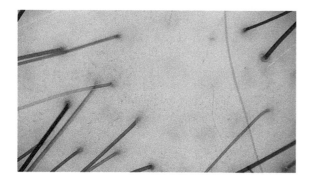

FIGURE 24.5 Irregularly distributed comma vessels in SD (×60).

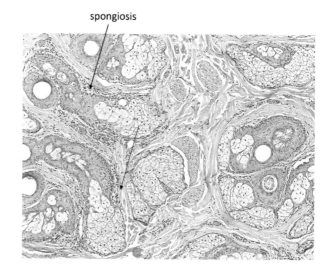

FIGURE 24.8 Spongiosis in the follicular epithelium.

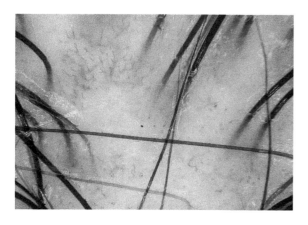

FIGURE 24.6 Linear loops (hairpin vessels) in SD (×70). (Courtesy to Giselle Martins, MD.)

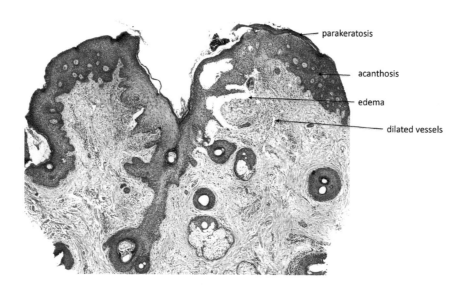

FIGURE 24.9 Irregular acanthosis with shoulder parakeratosis, edema in the papillary dermis and mild perivascular lymphocytic infiltrate around dilated vessels.

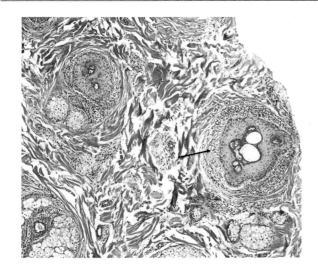

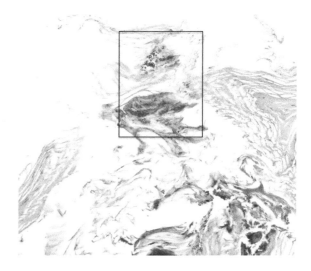

FIGURE 24.10 Perifollicular lymphohistiocytic infiltrate at the infundibular level in SD. Note the edema in the connective tissue sheath (arrow). There is no concentric perifollicular fibrosis and there is no consumption of the follicular epithelium as observed in scarring alopecia.

FIGURE 24.12 *Malassezia* spores in the stratum corneum (PAS stain).

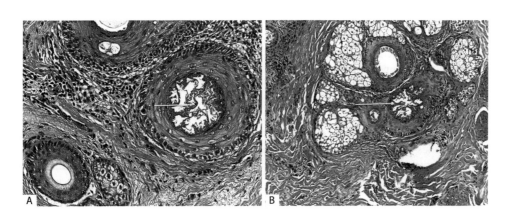

FIGURE 24.11 (A, B) Dilated sebaceous canal in SD (arrow), spongiosis and inflammatory infiltrate in the dermis.

FURTHER READING

Belew PW, Rosenberg EW, Jennings BR. Activation of the alternative pathway of complement by malassezia ovalis (pityrosporum ovale). Mycopathologia. 1980 Mar 31;70(3):187–91 https://emedicine.medscape.com/article/1108312-overview#a6

Kim GW, Jung HJ, Ko HC, Kim MB, Lee WJ, Lee SJ, et al. (2011) Dermoscopy can be useful in differentiating scalp psoriasis from seborrhoeic dermatitis. Br J Dermatol. 164(3):652–6.

Rudnicka, L, Oszewska M, Rakowska A, eds. *Atlas of Trichoscopy – Dermoscopy in Hair and Scalp Disease.* 1st ed. London: Springer-Verlag; 2012:371–378

Wikramanayake TC, Borda LJ, Miteva M, Paus R. Seborrheic dermatitis—Looking beyond *Malassezia.* Exp Dermatol. 2019 Sep;28(9):991–1001.

Red Scalp Disease*

25

Contents

Red scalp disease (RSD) or red scalp syndrome was first described by Thestrup-Pedersen in 1987 and only few reports since then can be found in the literature. However, the prevalence in the trichology practice may actually be higher as cases are most likely underdiagnosed and underreported due to lack of diagnostic criteria. RSD presents with sensitive, itchy or more often burning scalp, erythema, prominent vascular pattern and/or red papules, or pustules that cannot be attributed to any other diagnostic category after a complete work up has been completed. Of note, it does not respond to treatment with topical steroids or antiseborrheic drugs.

GENERAL CONCEPTS

- Patents complain of *sensitive*—itchy or more often burning scalp, that is particularly sensitive in some areas ("hot spots") and usually worse in the sun (Figure 25.1).
- Associated rosacea on the face is present in about at least half of the patients (personal observation) and one should always examine the face as many patients are unaware of its presence when asymptomatic; the dermoscopic finding of linear vessels arranged horizontally and vertically in a polygonal pattern is considered highly sensitive for erythematotelangiectatic rosacea (ER) and can be detected using a handheld dermatoscope (Figure 25.2).

- On *clinical exam,* the scalp shows (1) erythema that is more visible in patients with androgenetic alopecia (AGA) (Figure 25.3). According to some authors, majority of the patients have AGA, leading to speculations over the role of chronic ultraviolet (UV) light exposure. In fact, photodamaged skin is characterized by epidermal and dermal thinning and telangiectasia. However, the vessels do not form the characteristic polygonal pattern; (2) follicular papules and pustules (Figure 25.3); (3) fine scale.
- Many patients complain of increased shedding.
- Complete work up should include trichoscopy, pathology (I usually take two scalp biopsies for vertical sections from the most sensitive area of the scalp), serology panel to exclude a connective tissue disease, x-ray of the cervical spine (or MRI, or CT to exclude degenerative disk disease, anterolisthesis, osteophytes, lordosis, kyphosis and nerve root impingement), thorough work up for chronic pruritus including hematologic work up and patch test for contact dermatitis (standard series and cosmetic series); if pustules are present, a microbial culture should be obtained for completeness and to rule out gram negative folliculitis.
- Discontinuation of topical steroids and initiation of oral doxycycline leads to improvement of the symptoms in most patients.
- On *trichoscopy,* the most prominent pattern is the vascular pattern—a polarized videodermoscope at high magnification (>50×) allows to appreciate: (1) dilated and tortuous vessels of both polygonal and arborizing patterns (Figures 25.4–25.6); the arborizing pattern appears to be more distinct from seborrheic dermatitis as the most repetitive feature is a thicker linear vessel with numerous shorter and

* Special acknowledgement is due to Camila Jaramillo, MS, for contributing to the Trichoscopy section and to Giselle Martins, MD, for contributing to the concept.

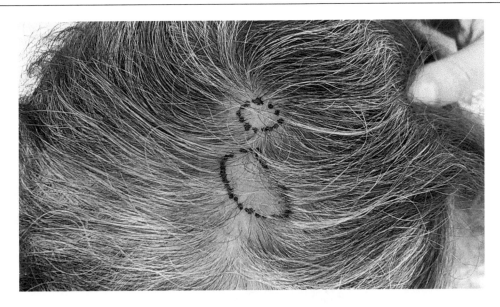

FIGURE 25.1 This patient with RSD pointed at the most sensitive areas of the scalp.

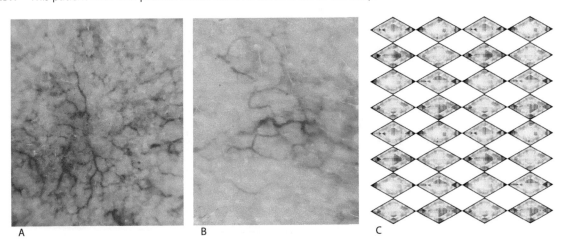

A   B   C

FIGURE 25.2 (A, B) Two patients with erythematotelangiectatic rosacea showed (C) rhomboid polygons on the cheeks (×20). Note the white scale in (B), representing *Demodex* tails.

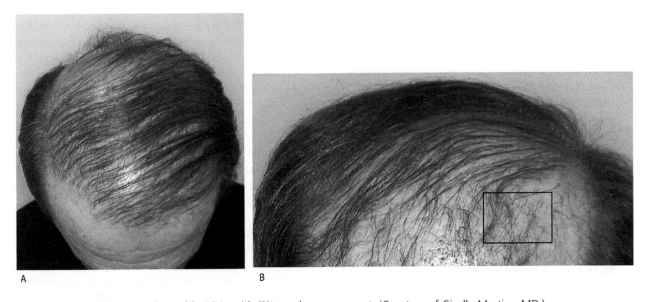

A   B

FIGURE 25.3 (A) RSD in a patient with AGA, with (B) papular component. (Courtesy of Giselle Martins, MD.)

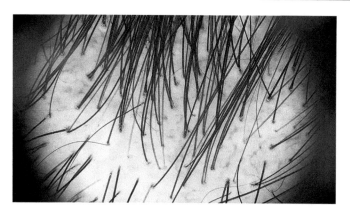

FIGURE 25.4   RSD showing abnormal vessels in a similar rhomboid polygons like pattern (see Figure 25.2) (×40).

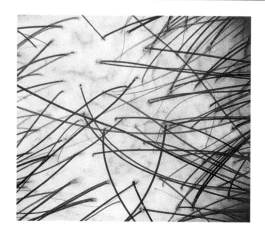

FIGURE 25.5   Arborizing vessels organized in a network (×40).

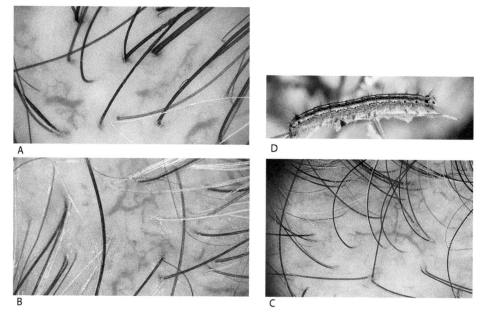

FIGURE 25.6   (A, B, C) Three more examples of arborizing vessels that form a network (×50). The vessels have a common pattern of thin ramifications coming out of a thicker linear trunk, resembling (D) caterpillar hair.

thinner ramifications along its length resembling *caterpillar hair* (Figure 25.6); (2) white-yellow greasy scales with an elongated shape at the site of the follicular ostia or in interfollicular proximity which most likely correspond to cones of infundibular parakeratosis or mounds of interfollicular parakeratosis (Figure 25.7) and (3) folliculocentric pustules and diffuse erythema (Figure 25.8).

MAIN HISTOLOGIC FEATURES

- Normal epidermis with basket weave stratum corneum in the vertical sections and the uppermost horizontal sections (Figure 25.9) but mounds of infundibular parakeratosis can be seen in cases with scaling (Figure 25.7).

- The upper dermis appears pale due to accumulation of edema (Figure 25.9), which may vary from slight to pronounced edema that separates the collagen bundles (Figures 25.10 and 25.11).
- The pilosebaceous structures are intact with hyperplastic or normal sebaceous glands (Figure 25.9).
- Dilated vessels are prominent in the upper dermis and there is mild perivascular and interstitial lymphocytic and mast cell infiltrate (Figures 25.9–25.12).
- *Demodex* mites maybe present in the follicular canals in about a third of the cases.
- Mild perivascular and perifollicular lymphocytic infiltrate with mast cells and individual eosinophils (Figure 25.13).
- In cases with pustules, the neutrophil collections are centered on the infundibula (not along the entire follicular length compared to folliculitis).

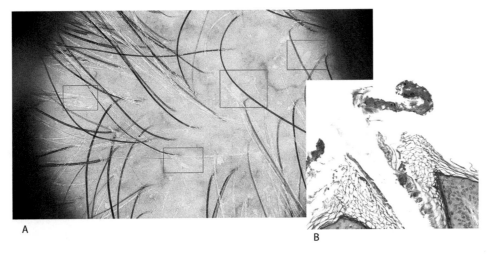

FIGURE 25.7   (A) White-yellow greasy scale with elongated shape (cone-like shape) at the follicular ostia but also in interfollicular distribution (×40), corresponding to (B) cones of parakeratosis centered on the follicular infundibula.

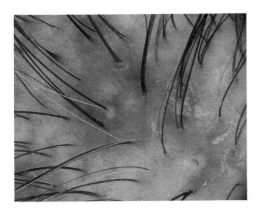

FIGURE 25.8   Pustules and diffuse erythema in RSD (×50). (Courtesy of Giselle Martins, MD.)

PEARLS

- *RSD is a diagnosis of exclusion.*
- Always perform a complete work-up as suggested above and look at the central face for features of rosacea – dermoscopy can be invaluable tool to detect the polygonal rhomboid structures.

FURTHER READING

Cribier B. Rosacea under the microscope: characteristic histological findings. J Eur Acad Dermatol Venereol. 2013 Nov;27(11):1336–43.

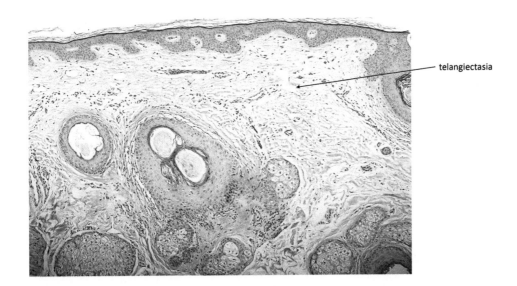

FIGURE 25.9   RSD shows normal stratum corneum, edema in the upper dermis (pale dermis) and dilated vessels; the sebaceous glands are of normal size. There is mild perifollicular and interstitial infiltrate of lymphocytes, mast cells and occasional eosinophils.

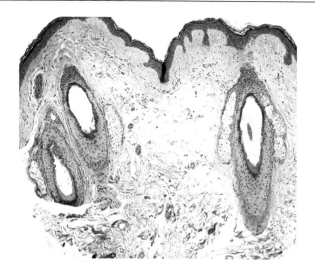

FIGURE 25.10   Significant dermal edema in a case of RSD. Note the normal epidermis and the solar elastosis in the dermis (the sebaceous glands are hypoplastic because this is a biopsy from an elderly patient).

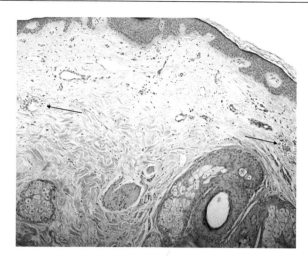

FIGURE 25.12   Note the dilated blood vessels and the edema in the dermis. There is also focal red blood cell extravasation (arrows).

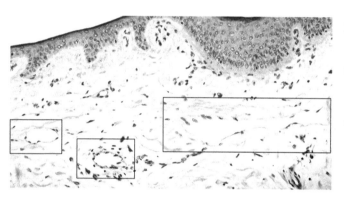

FIGURE 25.11   Telangiectasia and pronounced dermal edema in RSD.

Lallas A, Argenziano G, Apalla Z, et al. Dermoscopic patterns of common facial inflammatory skin diseases. J Eur Acad Dermatol Venereol. 2013;28(5):609–614. doi:10.1111/jdv.12146.

Oberholzer PA, Nobbe S, Kolm I, Kerl K, Kamarachev J, Trüeb RM. Red scalp disease—a rosacea-like dermatosis of the scalp? Successful therapy with oral tetracycline. Dermatology. 2009;219(2):179–81.

Thestrup-Pedersen K, Hjorth N: Red scalp: a previously undescribed disease of the scalp? Ugeskr Laeger 1987;149:2141–2142.

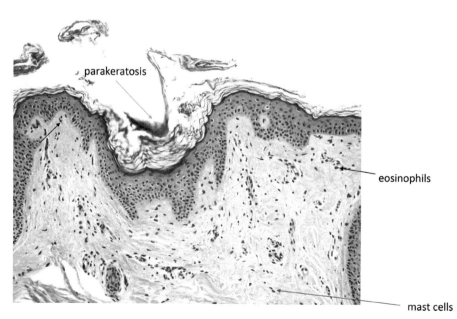

FIGURE 25.13   RSD shows a cone of parakeratosis in the follicular ostium and otherwise normal epidermis; note the eosinophils and mast cells in the dermis.

Scalp Involvement in Dermatomyositis

26

Contents

Dermatomyositis (DM) is an idiopathic inflammatory myopathy with classic cutaneous findings such as Gottron's papules of the hands and a heliotrope rash around the eyes, poikiloderma in a photosensitive distribution on the upper back, and V sign on the neck and chest, and periungual changes including hyperkeratotic, ragged cuticles, periungual erythema, capillary loss, and also irregularly enlarged and bushy capillaries with hemorrhage. Scalp involvement is commonly seen in DM and presents as a diffuse, erythematous, scaly, atrophic dermatosis with the common symptoms being burning, pruritus or *burning pruritus*.

GENERAL CONCEPTS

- The most common scalp involvement in DM is psoriasiform dermatitis and therefore the main misdiagnosis is psoriasis or seborrheic dermatitis.
- Other scalp involvements include violaceous erythema, atrophy and non-scarring diffuse alopecia of telogen effluvium type (33–87.5%) (Figure 26.1).
- Scalp pruritus is usually accompanied by burning sensation (burning pruritus) and its severity correlates with the disease activity.
- Scalp pruritus is more common in anti-TIF-1γ antibody positive patients and since the latter is associated with malignancy, scalp pruritus in DM may be a paraneoplastic marker.

- A recent work has shown that scalp pruritus in DM can be of neuropathic etiology as scalp biopsies have demonstrated features of small fiber neuropathy.
- On *trichoscopy,* there are: (1) enlarged tortuous capillaries and bushy capillaries that have been shown to correlate with the nail capillaroscopic findings (Figures 26.2 and 26.3); (2) peripilar casts (Figure 26.2); (3) interfollicular and perifollicular pigmentation, which corresponds to the pigment

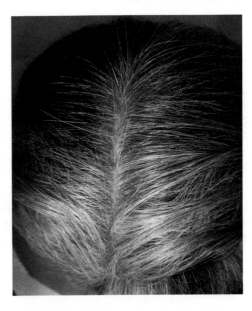

FIGURE 26.1 Violaceous erythema on the scalp in a patient with DM. (Courtesy of Julio Jasso, MD.)

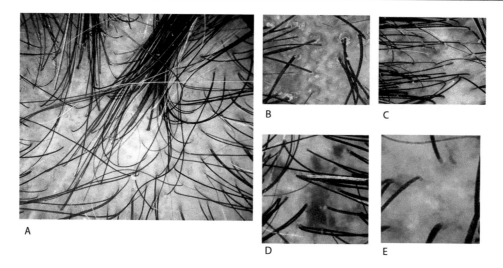

FIGURE 26.2 (A) Tortuous capillaries in scalp involvement in DM, (B) with peripilar casts, (C) interfollicular hyperpigmentation, (D) vascular lake-like structures, and (E) paleness of the scalp (×20). (Courtesy of Julio Jasso, MD.)

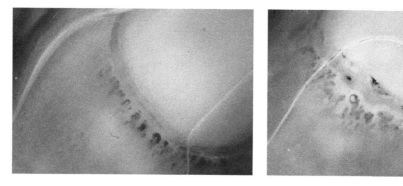

FIGURE 26.3 Nail capillaroscopy shows enlarged and bushy capillaries correlating with the similar vascular pattern on the scalp in DM (×20). (Courtesy of Julio Jasso, MD.)

incontinence from the interface dermatitis (Figure 26.2); (4) vascular lake-like structures (Figure 26.2) and (5) paleness of the scalp (Figure 26.2).

MAIN HISTOLOGIC FEATURES

Vertical sections remain the preferred mode of specimen bisection for scalp involvement in DM although the findings have been characterized on horizontal sections.

Vertical Sections

- Moderate-to-significant deposition of mucin in the papillary dermis, which corresponds to the paleness of the skin observed on dermoscopy (Figures 26.2 and 26.4).

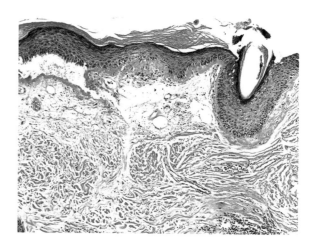

FIGURE 26.4 DM shows pronounced edema and mucin in the upper dermis. Note also the interface dermatitis with thickened basement membrane.

- Numerous abnormally dilated capillaries, some of them reaching length up to 1 mm, mostly in the papillary dermis but also in the reticular dermis.
- Epidermal atrophy and hyperkeratosis (Figure 26.5).
- Interface dermatitis ranging from focal vacuolar damage with pigment incontinence (Figure 26.6) to continuous detachment of the epidermis from the dermis forming a broad cleft due to the significant vacuolar damage (Figure 26.4).
- Thickened basement membrane, characterized as thick homogenous pink outline of the epidermis

that can be either segmental (50%) or focal (35%) (Figure 26.7).
- Lymphocytic infiltrate as individual clusters of lymphocytes or more commonly as patchy perivascular and perifollicular infiltrate; it extends occasionally along the eccrine ducts (Figure 26.8).
- Neutrophils can be observed mostly as individual cells and nuclear dust in the papillary dermis among the mucin strands; eosinophils can be observed as individual cells throughout the dermis and in perifollicular distribution (Figure 26.9).

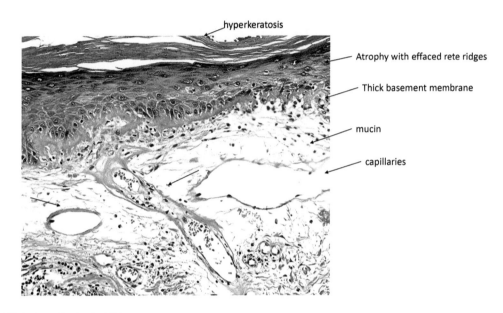

FIGURE 26.5   Dilated capillaries in DM.

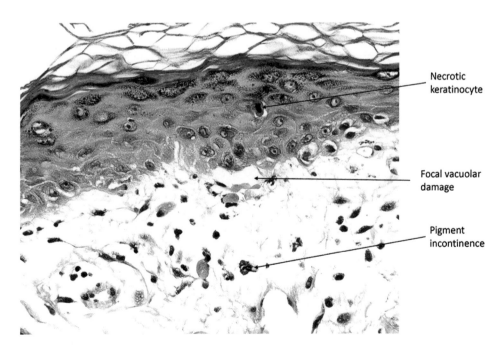

FIGURE 26.6   Interface dermatitis in DM.

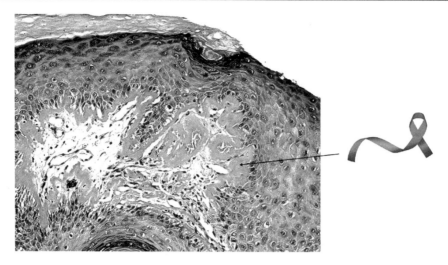

FIGURE 26.7   (A) Segmental thick basement membrane (arrow) like (B) "pink ribbon".

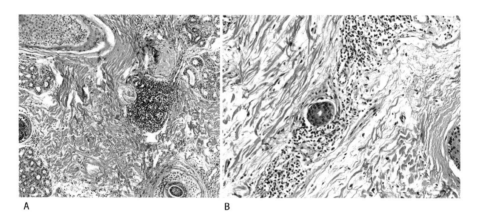

FIGURE 26.8   The lymphocytic infiltrate shows a patchy perivascular (B), lymphoid follicle-like aggregates (A) and extends occasionally along eccrine ducts (B).

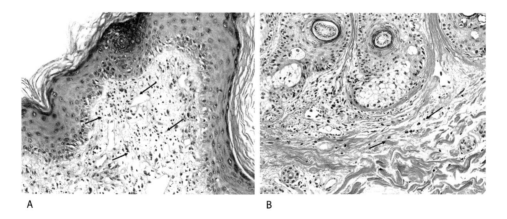

FIGURE 26.9   Neutrophils with (A) nuclear dust and (B) eosinophils in a specimen of scalp involvement in DM.

- Preservation of the sebaceous glands in majority of the cases (see Horizontal Sections).
- Unusual findings include acrosyringeal hypergranulosis (70%) (Figures 26.9A and 26.10), infundibular hypergranulosis (45%) (Figure 26.7) and focal parakeratosis (20%).

Horizontal Sections

Additional features in horizontal sections include:

- Mucin in the upper dermis appreciated as pale loose stroma among the follicular units at the level of the isthmus and above; forming a "mucinous mantle"

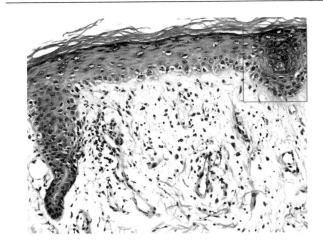

FIGURE 26.10   Acrosyringeal hypergranulosis.

(20% of the specimens) – the mucin appears as a mantle of loose pale stroma with dispersed lymphocytic infiltrate around individual follicular units (Figure 26.11).

- Interface dermatitis presents as vacuolar changes of the basal layer of the follicular epithelium at the level of the isthmus and the infundibulum (Figure 26.12).
- A thickened undulating basement membrane outlines as a pink ribbon the follicular epithelium in 50% of the cases (Figure 26.12).

- Overall preserved follicular architecture with regularly distributed follicular units (average of 11) containing sebaceous glands in 81%; a small percentage of cases may show sebaceous gland atrophy as mantle-like structures at the level of the isthmus (Figure 26.13).
- The average follicular density is reduced to 19.7 follicles with a terminal:vellus ratio of 4:1 and a telogen count 10.3%.

PEARLS

- In patients with violaceous, atrophic psoriasiform dermatitis and burning pruritus always rule out DM.
- Scalp itch in DM could be a clue to paraneoplastic DM.
- Dermal mucin, including in perifollicular distribution (as a mantle), and telangiectasia are almost universally present in scalp biopsies from scalp involvement in DM.
- The alopecia is non-scarring, with reduced follicular density and, on horizontal sections, the follicular counts are most consistent with the diagnosis of chronic telogen effluvium.

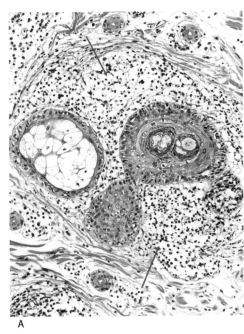
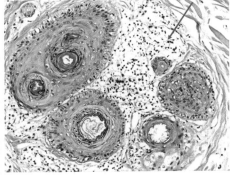

FIGURE 26.11   (A, B) Perifollicular mucinous mantle in scalp involvement in DM (loose pale stroma with dispersed lymphocytic infiltrate around individual follicular units).

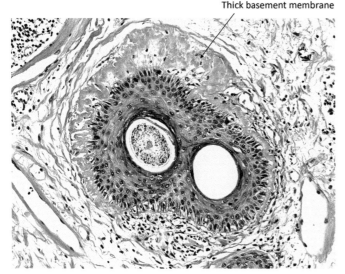

Thick basement membrane

FIGURE 26.12 Interface dermatitis of the follicular epithelium at the isthmus level. Note the thick undulation "pink ribbon-like" basement membrane.

FURTHER READING

Callen JP. Dermatomyositis. Lancet. 2000;355(9197):53–57.

Cassano N, Amerio P, D'Ovidio R, Vena GA. Hair disorders associated with autoimmune connective tissue diseases. G Ital Dermatol Venereol. 2014;149:555–65.

Jasso-Olivares J, Diaz-Gonzalez JM, Miteva M. Horizontal and vertical sections of scalp biopsy specimens from dermatomyositis patients with scalp involvement. J Am Acad Dermatol. 2018 Jun;78(6):1178–84.

Jasso-Olivares JC, Tosti A, Miteva M, Domminguez-Cherit J, Diaz-Gonzalez JM. Clinical and dermoscopic features of the scalp in 31 patients with dermatomyositis. Skin Appendage Disord. 2017;3:119–24.

Lee, N, Yosipovitch G. The itchy scalp. In Miteva M, ed. *Alopecia.*, 1st ed. Elsevier, 2018: 219–28.

Trueb RM. Involvement of scalp and nails in lupus erythematosus. Lupus. 2010;19(9):1078–86.

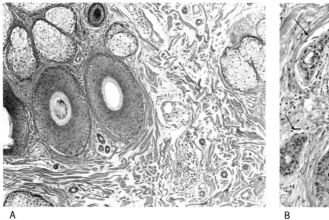
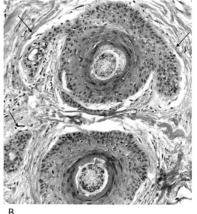

A   B

FIGURE 26.13   (A) Intact sebaceous glands in majority of the cases and (B) atrophic sebaceous glands in a small percentage of cases.

Linear Morphea
En Coup De Sabre

27

Contents

Linear morphea *en coup de sabre* (LMECDS) is a type of morphea that involves the scalp in a linear pattern resulting in atrophic scarring alopecia that resembles the shape of the cut from a sword.

GENERAL CONCEPTS

- LMECDS usually affects young individuals (83% of the patients are under the age of 25).
- It follows Blaschko's lines and presents as slightly elevated erythematous plaque that evolves into a vertical linear white shiny plaque adjacent the midline of the frontal scalp and forehead. The cicatricial alopecia and the skin involvement usually do not extend beyond the eyebrow (Figure 27.1).
- Variations include: two lines either on the same side or bilaterally, three lines on the same side, involvement of the vertex, and occiput.
- Unusual presentation includes an atrophic patch on the posterior vertex where Blaschko's lines have a spiral configuration (Figure 27.2), which usually transforms into a linear plaque eventually.
- The differential diagnosis for LMECDS includes linear lesions of lupus erythematosus, lichen planopilaris and erosive pustular dermatosis of the scalp, and histology can help make that distinction.
- On *trichoscopy,* the following features have been described: loss of follicular openings on a whitish

skin surface; scattered black dots, broken hairs, and pili torti like hairs; and short thick linear and branching tortuous vessels in the periphery of the lesion simulating those in lupus erythematosus (Figure 27.3A); fibrotic beams and small whitish patches (Figure 27.3B).

MAIN HISTOLOGIC FEATURES

- On *vertical sections,* the specimen appears square (the cookie cutter sign) due to the most pronounced finding which is dermal sclerosis (thickened and homogenized pink collagen that fills the entire dermis) (Figure 27.4).
  - Atrophy and entrapment of the eccrine glands in the sclerotic collagen (they lose their fat pad and are misplaced in the dermis instead of the dermo-subdermal border) (Figure 27.5)
  - Collagenous replacement of the adipose tissue
  - Absence of sebaceous glands but preservation of the arrector pili muscles (Figure 27.5)
  - Columnar and slender atrophic epithelial structures from follicular origin (Figures 27.6 and 27.7); these structures most likely arise from the compressing effect of the sclerotic stroma on the follicle resulting in hair cycle arrest
- *Horizontal sections* reveal a specimen with a strikingly well delineated oval/round shape (the cookie cutter sign but in the transverse plane) (Figure 27.8).

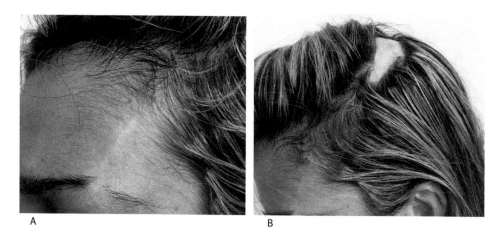

FIGURE 27.1   (A, B) Linear morphea *en coup de sabre* extending to the left eyebrow in a young woman. (Courtesy of Rodrigo Pirmez, MD.)

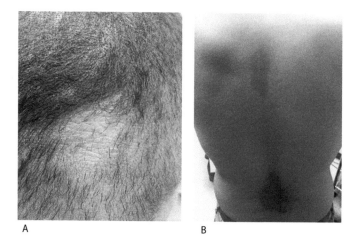

FIGURE 27.2   (A) A round patch of burnt out morphea on posterior scalp and (B) aligned with two patches along the midline of the back.

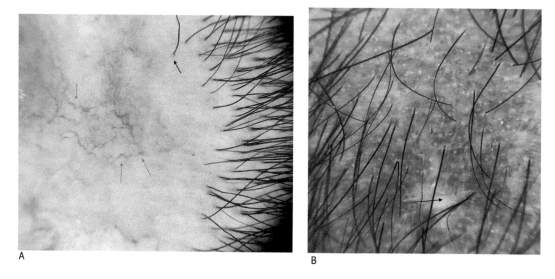

FIGURE 27.3   (A) Dermoscopy shows branching tortuous vessels (blue arrows) and pili torti-like hairs (black arrows) at the periphery of the lesion. (Courtesy of Rodrigo Pirmez, MD.) (B) In a case of burnt out morphea, there are white fibrotic beams (blue arrows) and small whitish patches (black arrows); note also the broken hairs (×20).

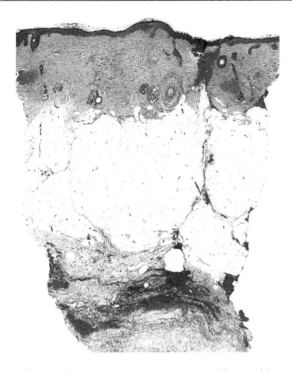

FIGURE 27.4 The specimen appears square (the cookie cutter sign) due to pronounced dermal sclerosis. Note the misplaced sweat coils in the dermis.

- Atrophic epithelial structures from follicular origin that resemble telogen germinal units in the horizontal sections (Figure 27.9).
- Perineural lymphocytic and plasmocytic infiltrate extending into the subcutis and fascia may also be present (perineural inflammation in skin lesions of morphea can be identified in at least half of the cases) (Figure 27.10).

PEARLS

- Early cases (especially cut as horizontal sections) can mimic subacute stage alopecia areata due to the increased number of telogen germinal units like structures. In such cases, the sharp outline of the specimen, the entrapment of the sweat coils and the strikingly pink stroma composed of thick collagen bundles are clues to LMECDS (Figure 27.11).

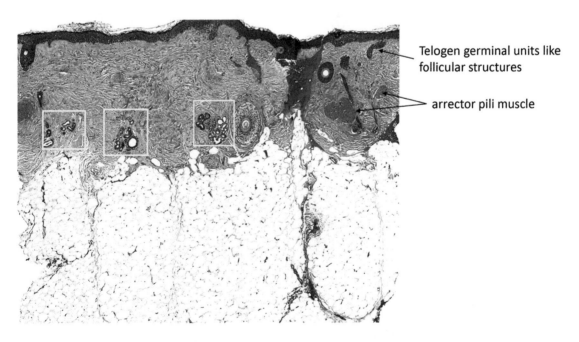

Telogen germinal units like follicular structures

arrector pili muscle

FIGURE 27.5 The sweat coils are placed in the reticular dermis; they show atrophy and absence of the fat pad.

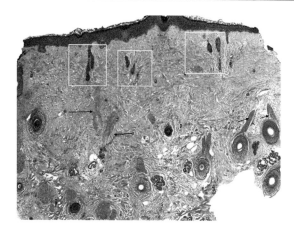

FIGURE 27.6 Atrophic follicular epithelial structures (quadrants), solitary arrector pili muscles (arrows), and misplaced sweat coils in the thick sclerotic stroma.

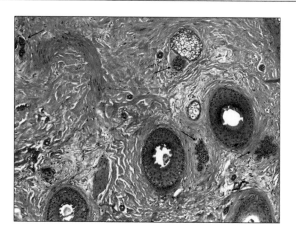

FIGURE 27.7 Telogen germinal units like follicular structures (black arrows) and arector pili muscle (yellow arrow).

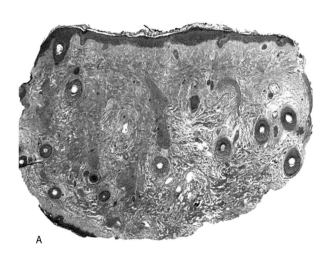

A

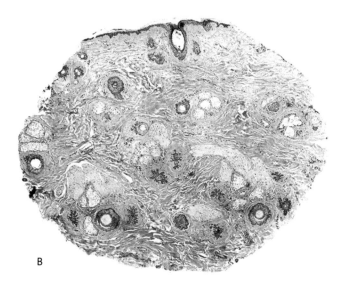

B

FIGURE 27.8 (A, B) Horizontal sections of scalp biopsies from linear morphea *en coup de sabre* show a sharp oval shape due to the retraction of the sclerotic stroma.

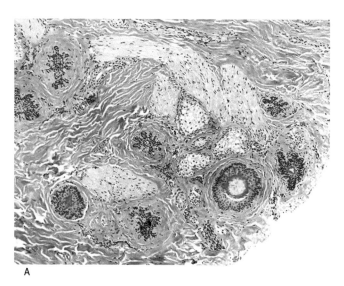

A

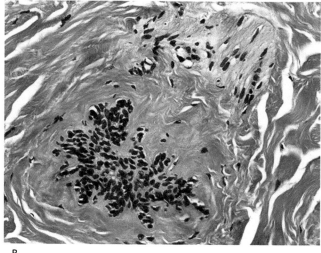

B

FIGURE 27.9 (A, B) Telogen germinal units like structures in a case of linear morphea.

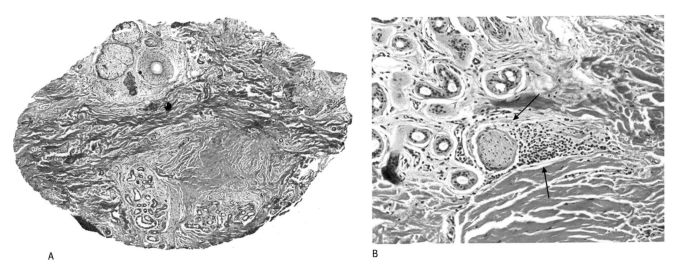

A   B

FIGURE 27.10   (A) Another example shows the sharp oval outline, sclerotic stroma, entrapment of the sweat coils, and telogen germinal unit like structure. (B) Note the perineural lymphocytic infiltrate.

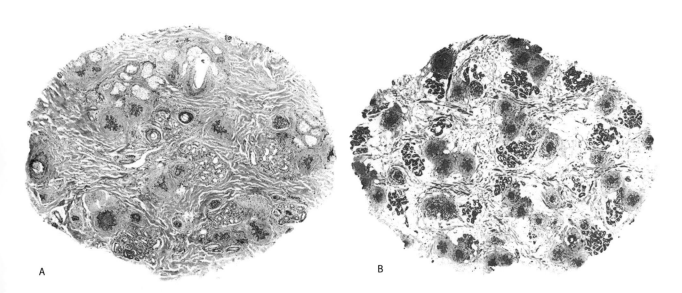

A   B

FIGURE 27.11   (A) Horizontal sections of early stage linear morphea *en coup de sabre* can mimic (B) alopecia areata on low power.

FURTHER READING

Goh C, Biswas A, Goldberg LJ. Alopecia with perineural lymphocytes: a clue to linear scleroderma en coup de sabre. J Cutan Pathol. 2012;39:518–520.

Pierre-Louis M, Sperling LC, Wilke MS, Hordinsky MK. Distinctive histopathologic findings in linear morphea (en coup de sabre) alopecia. J Cutan Pathol. 2013;40:580–584

Saceda-Corralo D, Nusbaum AG, Romanelli P, Miteva M. A case of circumscribed scalp morphea with perineural lymphocytes on pathology. Skin Appendage Disord. 2017;3:175–178.

Saceda-Corralo D, Tosti A. Trichoscopic features of linear morphea on the scalp. Skin Appendage Disord. 2018;4(1):31–33. doi:10.1159/000478022

Hair and Scalp Infections

28

Contents

TINEA CAPITIS

Tinea capitis (TC) is a contagious dermatophyte infection of the scalp and the hair.

GENERAL CONCEPTS

- There are two main causative pathogens in TC: *Trichophyton* (anthropophilic) and *Microsporum* (zoophilic).
- The type of hair invasion is classified as ectothrix (the dermatophytes grow inside the follicle and the fungal spores cover the outside of the hair shaft whose cuticle is destroyed), endothrix (the dermatophyte invades and grows within the hair shaft and the fungal spores remain in the hair shaft and the cuticle is intact) or favus (clusters of hyphae at the base of the hairs, with air spaces in the hair shafts giving rise to the characteristic cup-shaped yellow crusts known as scutula). Ectothrix infections

(*M. canis*) potentially spread rapidly whereas endothrix (*T. tonsurans*) and favic infections (*T. shoenleini*) are less contagious.

- TC most commonly affects pre-pubertal children; in the United States, it is most common in female children, and in 95% is caused by *T. tonsurans*. *M. canis* is the predominant causative organism in many countries of the Mediterranean basin.
- The three most common clinical patterns are: (1) *non-inflammatory black dot pattern*: hairless patches with black dots in the alopecic patch due to hair breakage at or below the scalp surface due to endothrix infection; it clinically simulates alopecia areata and trichotillomania (Figure 28.1A,B); (2) *non-inflammatory seborrheic dermatitis pattern*: diffuse or focal, fine, white, adherent scale affecting the scalp without alopecia which resembles dandruff (Figure 28.1C); (3) *Kerion celsi or inflammatory tinea capitis* – one or multiple tender, inflamed and boggy, alopecic nodules with pustules on their surface which have the potential to evolve into scarring alopecia (Figure 28.1D). Some cases may be indistinguishable from dissecting cellulitis

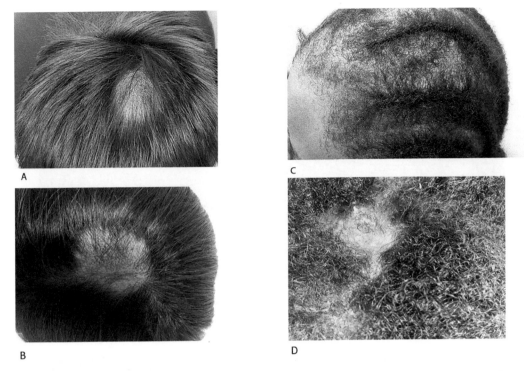

FIGURE 28.1 The three clinical patterns of tinea capitis: (A, B) two examples of non-inflammatory black dot pattern, (C) non-inflammatory seborrheic dermatitis pattern, and (D) inflammatory tinea capitis (kerion).

of the scalp (*Tinea capitis mimicking dissecting cellulitis*), especially when this variant is often encountered in adults and clinically simulates folliculitis or dissecting cellulitis. Utilizing all work up tools such as KOH preparation, trichoscopy, histology or fungal culture is necessary to establish the correct diagnosis.

- On *trichoscopy*, the following hair shaft abnormalities have been described: broken hairs, corkscrew hairs, comma hairs, barcode hairs, zigzag hairs and black dots (Figures 28.2 and 28.3).
  - Comma hairs are specific for TC and are reported in both Caucasians and African Americans whereas corkscrew hairs are exclusive to African Americans but can be seen also in ectodermal dysplasia. Comma hairs are dark short hairs of uniform color, thickness and

sharp diagonal whereas circle hairs that can be seen in alopecia areata are thinner and longer, regularly twisted hairs with tapered ends (see Chapters 1 and 8).
  - Identifying comma hairs spares the need for the biopsy in young children (Figures 28.2 and 28.3).

MAIN HISTOLOGIC FEATURES

- In tinea capitis caused by ectothrix infection, the hyphae and spores cover the outside surface of the hair shaft, which results in destruction of the cuticle.

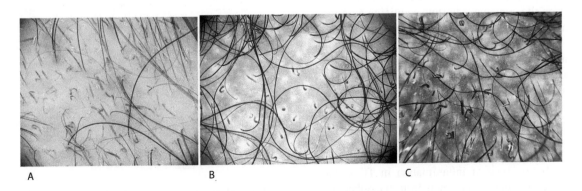

FIGURE 28.2 Examples of comma hairs in (A) a Caucasian boy and (B, C) two African American girls.

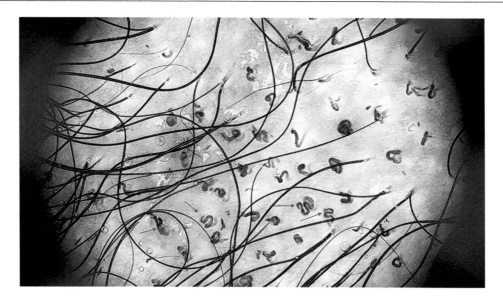

FIGURE 28.3   Broken, comma and corkscrew hairs (arrow) in an African American child.

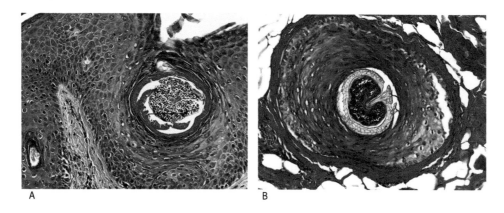

A   B

FIGURE 28.4   Fungal spores within the hair shaft: (A) note the intact cuticle (arrow). (B) The loaded hair shaft in African American hair bends further on the concave side acquiring a comma shape.

- In tinea capitis caused by endothrix infection, the inside of the hair shaft is invaded only by rounded and box like arthrospores and not by hyphae (Figures 28.4 and 28.7). In African American patients, the loaded shafts bend further on the concave side thus acquiring a comma shape on histology too (Figure 28.4).
- In inflammatory tinea capitis (kerion), there is a dense mixed cell inflammatory infiltrate of neutrophils, plasma cells, eosinophils, lymphocytes and histiocytes as well as giant cells (suppurative granulomatous folliculitis) (Figures 28.5 and 28.6). The special stains may be falsely negative in up to half of the cases and numerous sections are required in order to identify a positive hair shaft (Figure 28.7). The abscess type of inflammation in TC usually occupies the entire specimen from the subcutaneous fat to the infundibulum.

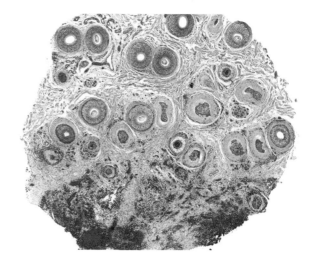

FIGURE 28.5   Inflammatory tinea capitis shows abscess-like dense inflammatory infiltrate and significant telogen shift.

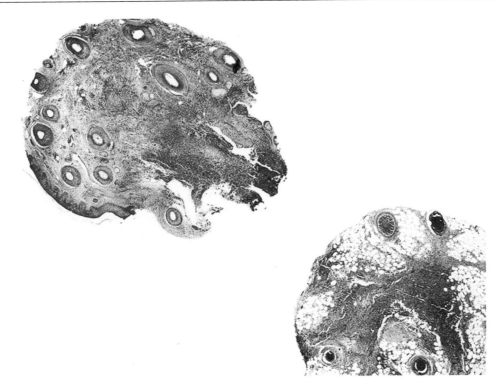

FIGURE 28.6 Another example of inflammatory tinea capitis showing the extent of inflammation from the subdermis to the epidermis.

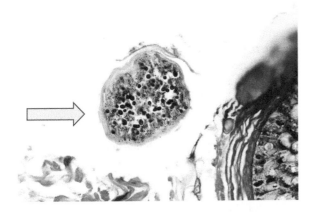

FIGURE 28.7 A single hair shaft is positive for fungal spores after numerous deeper sections have been cut and stained (PAS).

- Use a Wood's lamp examination of the scalp as an easy screening tool in TC: green fluorescence in *Microsporum* spp. vs. none in *Trichophyton* spp.
- In a biopsy submitted as rule out folliculitis vs. TC vs. dissecting cellulitis that shows significant inflammatory infiltrate, perform fungal stains and cut numerous sections (even through the block) in order to detect an affected hair shaft.

SYPHILIS

Syphilis is a systemic infectious disease caused by *Treponema pallidum*. Syphilitic alopecia (SA) is an uncommon clinical manifestation of secondary syphilis and can be the only manifestation of the disease.

PEARLS

- Comma hairs may be missing or difficult to find in inflammatory tinea capitis due to the heavy inflammation – look for them outside the boggy inflamed plaques and take the biopsy from there (Figure 28.8).

GENERAL CONCEPTS

- SA may clinically mimic a wide range of hair disorders, including alopecia areata, trichotillomania, lichen planopilaris, tinea capitis and telogen effluvium.

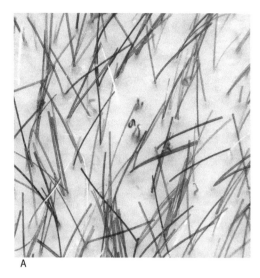

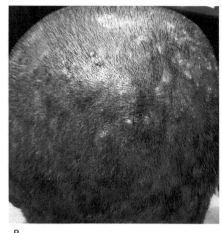

FIGURE 28.8   (A) A comma hair was found outside the boggy plaques and nodules in a case of kerion (B) and was selected as the site of the biopsy.

- SA is classified into two types:

1. *Symptomatic SA* presents with skin lesions on the scalp consistent with those encountered in secondary syphilis on the skin: these are usually papulosquamous lesions (Figure 28.9).
2. *Essential SA* is characterized by hair loss with no visible syphilitic lesions on the scalp; there are 3 variants (Figure 28.10):
   - Moth-eaten or patchy alopecia characterized by small alopecic patches irregularly distributed over the scalp
   - Diffuse alopecia, characterized by diffuse hair loss in a telogen effluvium-like pattern that can present at any time in the course of the infection and can also be one of the only early symptoms of syphilis
   - Mixed forms (combination of diffuse hair loss and alopecic moth-eaten patches)

- The diagnosis is established by serology (rapid plasma regain card test [RPR] and a *Treponema pallidum* hemagglutination test [TPHA]). Trichoscopy and pathology can be used as adjunct tools for the diagnosis but the features are largely non-specific.
- On *trichoscopy of moth-eaten SA,* there are:
  - Black dots, focal atrichia, hypopigmentation of the hair shafts and yellow dots in the center of the alopecic patches along with few black dots at the periphery (Figure 28.11a).
  - Some patients have reduction in the number of terminal hairs, which has been shown to be the main cause for the decreased hair density in the moth eaten pattern (Figure 28.11B).
  - Tapering hairs can be detected at the periphery of the moth-eaten patches as single or double bending.

MAIN HISTOLOGIC FEATURES

- The histology of the moth-eaten SA can be indistinguishable from acute stage alopecia areata.
- A reduced number of anagen follicles and an increased number of catagen and telogen follicles (which corresponds to the trichoscopic finding of reduced number of terminal follicles and/or black dots) (Figure 28.12).

FIGURE 28.9   Symptomatic SA: note the diffuse hair loss co-localized to the area of erythematous livedoid papules (lichen planus-like lesions). (Courtesy of Giselle Martins, MD.)

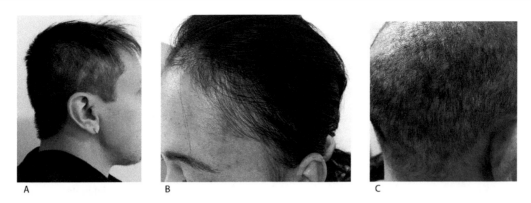

FIGURE 28.10   Essential SA presents with 3 subtypes: (A) moth-eaten patchy alopecia, (B) diffuse telogen effluvium-like alopecia, and (C) mixed – patchy and diffuse alopecia. (Courtesy of Giselle Martins, MD.)

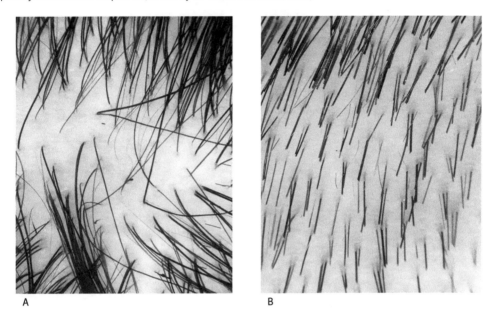

FIGURE 28.11   (A) Black dots at the periphery of a moth-eaten patch and (B) decreased number of terminal hairs (×20). (Courtesy of Giselle Martins, MD and Susana Ruiz-Tagle, MD.)

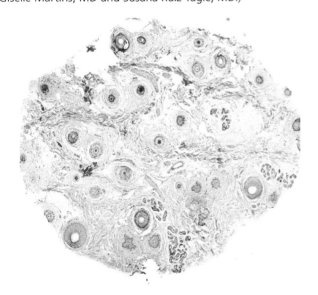

FIGURE 28.12   Moth-eaten SA shows increased telogen and vellus count.

- There is peribulbar lymphocytic infiltrate, widened infundibular ostia and pigmented casts (Figure 28.13).
- The presence of plasma cells in the infiltrate is not a sustainable finding for the diagnosis as they maybe absent or missed on the exam (Figure 28.14).

PEARLS

- The diagnosis can be suspected on pathology but since the findings can be indistinguishable from alopecia areata (moth-eaten alopecia pattern) or telogen effluvium (diffuse alopecia pattern), it requires a serologic confirmation.
- Plasma cells can be missing in 1/3 of the biopsies.
- Look in the fibrous streamers for plasma cells (Figure 28.14).

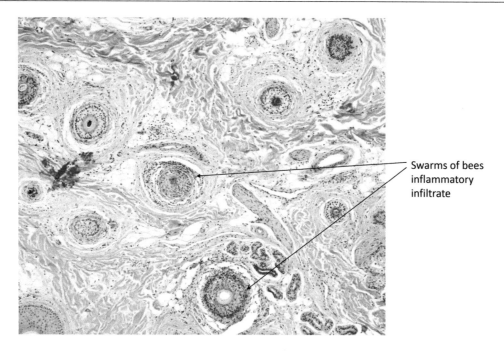

FIGURE 28.13   On higher power, swarm of bees infiltrate, similar to that observed in alopecia areata, can be detected.

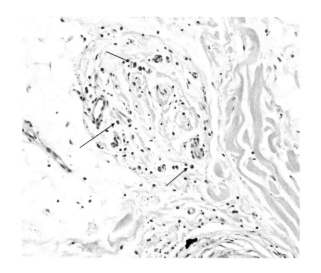

FIGURE 28.14   Plasma cells in fibrous streamers in moth-eaten SA.

HERPES ZOSTER

Herpes zoster (HZ) infection of the scalp can present as localized or dermatomal folliculitis and it can lead to associated non-scarring or scarring alopecia.

GENERAL CONCEPTS

- HZ on the scalp can present with erythematous papules, plaques *without vesicles and crusts* (in comparison to HZ on the skin) (Figure 28.15); a clue to the diagnosis is a dermatomal distribution respecting the midline and associated pain (unilateral otalgia in cases of Rumsey–Hunt syndrome).

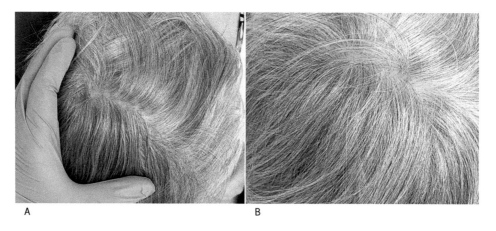

FIGURE 28.15   (A, B) Erythematous ill-defined plaques on the scalp sparing the midline in a patient with same side otalgia. Note the absence of blisters and crusts.

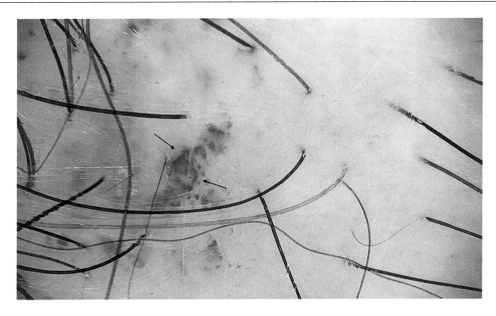

FIGURE 28.16 Dilated vessels with lakes of blood (black arrows) – compare with the normal loop-like vessels in the vicinity. There are empty dots (blue arrows) and yellow blotches (red arrows) (×50).

- Some studies have reported the association of alopecia areata (AA) and HZ infection – in some cases, the alopecia precedes the HZ infection and vice versa. A large population-based study from Taiwan reported that the odds for HZ infection are increased after a prior AA diagnosis within 3 years – the hypothesis behind this is that Varicella Zoster virus reactivation occurs due to an increased amount of inflammation and the high stress levels associated with AA patients.
- On *trichoscopy*, there are non-specific features of thick dilated vessels with lakes of blood (corresponding to the vasculitis-like changes), empty dots (corresponding to the necrotic follicular epithelium at the upper level) and yellow blotches (corresponding to the epidermal changes of ballooning keratinocyte degeneration) (Figure 28.16).

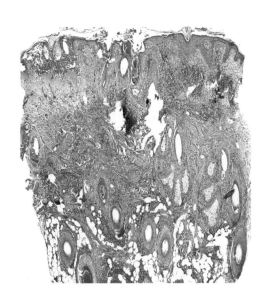

FIGURE 28.17 HZ on the scalp: intraepidermal blister and prominent superficial and deep perivascular and perifollicular inflammatory infiltrate.

MAIN HISTOLOGIC FEATURES

- Vertical sections are necessary for the diagnosis in order to allow the assessment of the epidermis.
- Intraepidermal blister with ballooned keratinocytes with slate gray nuclei, multinucleated acantholytic keratinocytes and necrosis ranging from individual necrotic kratinocytes to frank necrosis (Figures 28.17 and 28.18).
- Dense perifollicular and perivascular lymphocytic and neutrophilic infiltrate leading to leukocytoclastic vasculitis (Figures 28.17, 28.18 and 28.19).
- At its upper follicular levels, the follicular epithelium may show focal to complete necrosis – the

Varicella Zoster virus reaches the dermatome through the myelinated nerves which end around the isthmus of the hair follicles where the sebaceous glands enter (Figure 28.19).
- At its lower levels, the follicular epithelium does not show necrosis but a peribulbar "swarm of bees"-like infiltrate that closely resembles the findings in acute alopecia areata (Figure 28.20).
- The infiltrate can be noted also in perivascular or diffuse distribution, may surround the cutaneous nerves and cause a leukocytoclastic vasculitis (Figures 28.17–28.19).

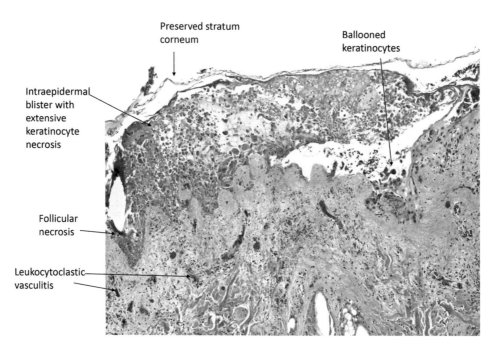

FIGURE 28.18   Typical HZ features on higher power.

- The Anti-Varicella Zoster virus immunohistochemistry antibody is strongly positive (Figure 28.19).

PEARLS

- Folliculosebaceous units are the first cutaneous epithelial structures to be targeted in HZ (this is why, early HZ can present with erythematous plaques only). In herpes simplex and varicella on the contrary, the epidermal involvement predominates at the onset (therefore, they always present with vesicles).

- As there is no vesicle/blister to perform a Tzanck prep, a scalp biopsy is crucial for the diagnosis. Other reported diagnostic tools in such cases include confocal microscopy, which can detect the ballooned keratinocytes in the lesions.

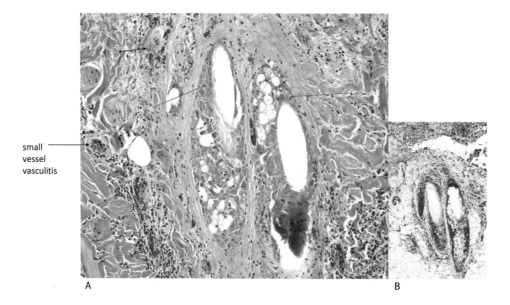

FIGURE 28.19   (A) Complete necrosis of the follicular epithelium and the sebaceous glands (red arrows); (B) the Anti-Varicella Zoster virus Immunohistochemistry Antibody is strongly positive.

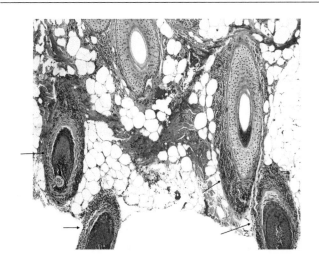

FIGURE 28.20 Peribulbar inflammation in HZ mimicking the swarm of bees infiltrate of alopecia areata.

FURTHER READING

Arenas R, Toussaint S, Isa-Isa R. Kerion and dermatophytic granuloma. Mycological and histopathological findings in 19 children with inflammatory tinea capitis of the scalp. Int J Dermatol. 2006;45:215–9.

Baek JH, Hong KC, Lee DY, Kim MS, Lee UH, Park HS. Alopecia areata associated with herpes zoster. J Dermatol. 2013;40(8):672.

Bi MY, Cohen PR, Robinson FW, Gray JM. Alopecia syphilitica – report of a patient with secondary syphilis presenting as moth-eaten alopecia and a review of its common mimickers. Dermatol Online J. 2009;15:6.

Boer A, Herder N, Winter K, Falk T. Herpes folliculitis: clinical, histopathological, and molecular pathologic observations. Br J Dermatol. 2006;154(4):743–6.

Chen CH, Wang KH, Hung SH, Lin HC, Tsai MC, Chung SD. Association between herpes zoster and alopecia areata: a population-based study. J Dermatol. 2015;42(8):824–5.

Lacarrubba F, Verzì AE, Musumeci ML, Micali G. Early diagnosis of herpes zoster by handheld reflectance confocal microscopy. J Am Acad Dermatol. 2015 Dec;73(6):e201–3.

Miletta NR, Schwartz C, Sperling L. Tinea capitis mimicking dissecting cellulitis of the scalp: a histopathologic pitfall when evaluating alopecia in the post-pubertal patient. J Cutan Pathol. 2014 Jan;41(1):2–4. doi: 10.1111/cup.12270.

Piraccini BM, Broccoli A, Starace M, et al. Hair and scalp manifestations in secondary syphilis: epidemiology, clinical features and trichoscopy. Dermatology. 2015;231(2):171–6.

Slowinska M, Rudnicka L, Schwartz RA, Kowalska-Oledzka E, Rakowska A, Sicinska J, et al. Comma hairs: a dermoscopic marker of tinea capitis: a rapid diagnostic method. J Am Acad Dermatol. 2008;59(5 Suppl):S77–9.

Miscellaneous

29

Contents

The goal of this chapter is to provide the reader with some helpful images and pearls about rare diagnoses encountered in the hair clinic and under the microscope, which are outside of the scope of the other chapters.

SARCOIDOSIS

Sarcoidosis is a systemic granulomatous disease that can rarely affect the scalp without other cutaneous lesions or systemic involvement.

- Clinically, the alopecia associated with sarcoidosis could be scarring or non-scarring and co-localizes to areas with erythema and scaling, indurated plaques and nodules (Figure 29.1).
- The lesions often resemble discoid lupus erythematosus or folliculitis.
- *Trichoscopy* shows *perifollicular and follicular yellowish to pale yellow orange round blotches* (Figure 29.2), decreased hair density, absence of follicular ostia, dystrophic hairs and telangiectasia.
- *Pathology* should be evaluated on vertical sections:
  - Sarcoidal granulomas consisting of epithelioid histiocytes surrounded by lymphocytes throughout the papillary and mid dermis are diagnostic; *lichenoid granulomas are a clue to sarcoidosis* (Figures 29.3 and 29.4).
  - Horizontal sections have been reported by others and reveal at the level of the isthmus

destruction of follicular units by granulomas and scattered miniaturized anagen follicles surrounded by epithelioid giant cells.
  - Birefringent foreign material has been described in up to 77% of the biopsies of cutaneous sarcoidosis and it has been postulated that foreign material may act as a nidus for granuloma formation (Figure 29.5).
- *Scalp sarcoidosis is often associated with systemic lung involvement.*
- *Search for other lesions on the face and the body as this can provide a clue to the diagnosis.*

AMYLOIDOSIS

Amyloidosis is characterized by the extracellular deposition of amyloid as monoclonal light-chain immunoglobulins in acquired systemic (AL) amyloidosis, non-immunoglobulinemic acute phase proteins in reactive systemic (AA) amyloidosis and in wild-type transthyretin amyloidosis.

- Alopecia in systemic amyloidosis can involve any hair bearing area and ranges from isolated non-scarring (patchy or diffuse) alopecia-to-alopecia universalis (Figure 29.6); all patients have some degree of plasma cell dyscrasia including multiple myeloma.
- *Trichoscopy* shows peripilar salmon-colored halos, which can be devoid of hair shafts or contain terminal and vellus hairs, black dots and/or broken hairs (Figure 29.7); the halo corresponds to the amyloid

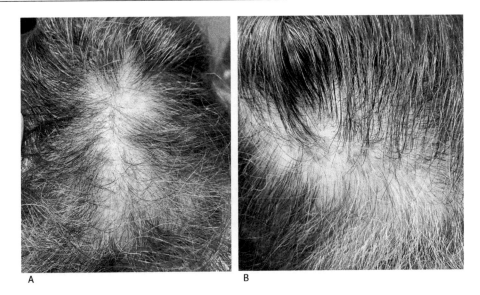

FIGURE 29.1 (A, B) Sarcoidosis on the scalp presents with orange macules and papules. The patient has concomitant androgenetic alopecia.

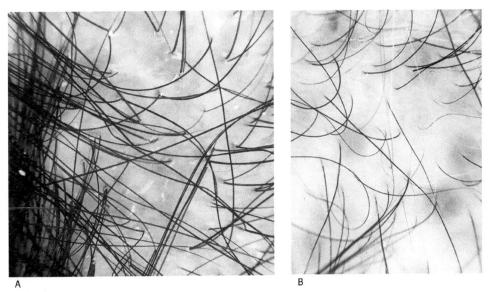

FIGURE 29.2 (A, B) Yellow-orange blotches on a background of diffuse erythema (×20) in two cases of sarcoidosis.

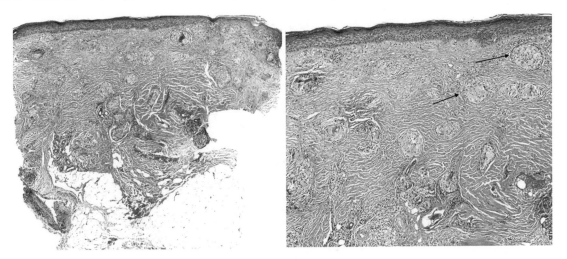

FIGURE 29.3 (A, B) Scalp sarcoidosis: lichenoid epithelioid granulomas.

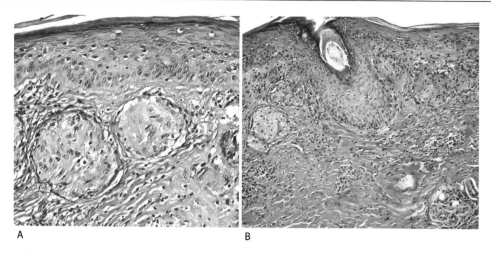

FIGURE 29.4 Sarcoidal granulomas in close apposition (A) to the dermo-epidermal junction and (B) to the follicular epithelium.

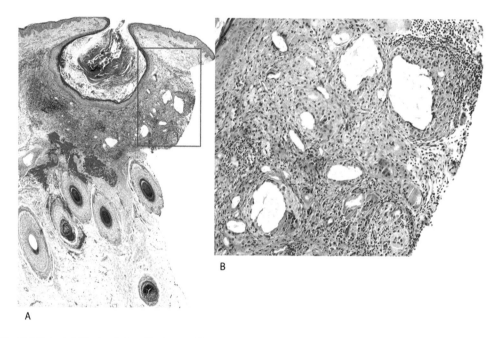

FIGURE 29.5 (A, B) Dilated follicular infundibulum with sarcoidal granulomas in a lichenoid pattern; note the birefringent foreign material within the granulomas.

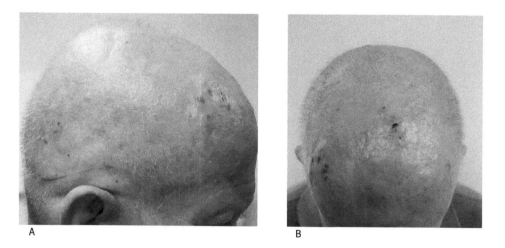

FIGURE 29.6 (A, B) Alopecia universalis in association with systemic amyloidosis in a patient with multiple myeloma.

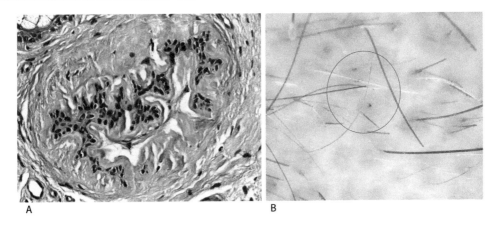

FIGURE 29.7 (A) The atrophic follicular structures compressed by the surrounding amyloid correspond to (B) the trichoscopic finding of dystrophic hairs surrounded by a salmon-colored halo.

deposited around the follicular structures leading to their atrophy and hair cycle arrest (Figure 29.7).

- *Pathology*
  - Horizontal sections: there is preserved follicular architecture with intact sebaceous glands (Figure 29.8).
  - Persistent telogen germinal units with only a few anagen follicles (as a sign of hair cycle arrest) similar to the ones seen in linear morphea *en coup de sabre* and permanent alopecia after chemotherapy (Figures 29.7 and 29.8)
  - Homogenous, eosinophilic deposits of amyloid surrounding follicular structures (Figure 29.9)

BRUNSTING-PERRY CICATRICIAL PEMPHIGOID OF THE SCALP

Brunsting-Perry cicatricial pemphigoid (BPCP) of the scalp is a rare disease – it is a type of mucous membrane pemphigoid (MMP) that was first described by Brunsting and Perry in 1957.

- BPCP occurs in 7% of the patients with MMP and almost exclusively spares the mucosa.
- Various target antigens have been recognized including: BP antigens 1 and 2 (BP230 and BP180),

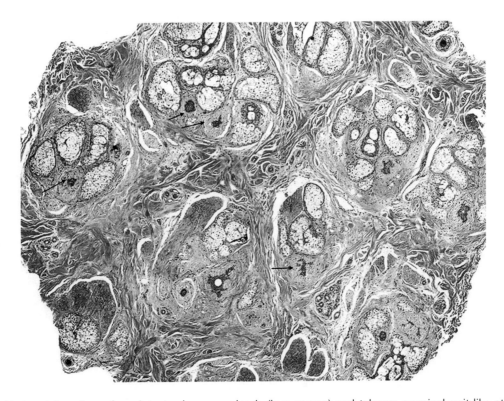

FIGURE 29.8 Horizontal sections show intact sebaceous glands (bue arrows) and telogen germinal unit-like atrophic follicular structures (black arrows).

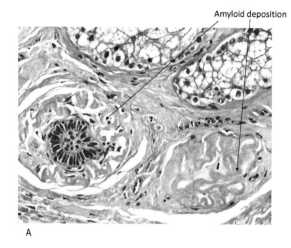

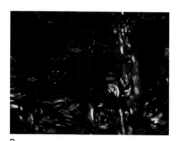

Amyloid deposition

B   Congo red under polarized light

A

FIGURE 29.9 (A) Mechanical constriction to the follicles caused by abnormal follicular or perifollicular deposition of amyloid (as highlighted in apple green by the congo red stain under polarized light in (B), collagen or mucin may lead eventually to anagen arrest.

laminin 5, laminin 332, laminin 311, type VII collagen and β4 integrin subunit.

- The clinical presentation is that of subepidermal blisters followed by scarring alopecia (Figures 29.10 and 29.11) as blistering in the scalp involving *lamina lucida and below* leads to scarring alopecia due to the inflammation in the upper portion of the hair follicle (the permanent portion of the follicle) and the interfollicular epidermis.
- However, BPCP causes alopecia in only a small subset of patients. The theories behind this selectiveness include lack of antibody-antigen target binding or ubiquitous binding with varying scarring responses between patients.
- *Trichoscopy* does not show specific features and is primarily helpful to rule out other types of scarring alopecia-like lichen planopilaris and folliculitis decalvans (Figure 29.11).

- *Direct immunofluorescence* from perileasional skin or from uninvolved buccal mucosa should be performed for the diagnosis – it confirms the linear deposition of IgG and C3 at the dermo-epidermal junction.
- *Pathology*
  - Subepidermal cleft (Figure 29.12)
  - Edema and variable, often lichenoid inflammatory infiltrate in the dermis (lymphocytes, histiocytes, plasma cells, eosinophils) and in perifollicular pattern with perifollicular fibrosis and lichenoid infiltrate at the isthmus level (Figures 29.12 and 29.13)
  - Absent sebaceous glands (Figure 29.13)
  - Dermal fibrosis (Figures 29.14 and 29.15)
  - The cleft could be taken for an artifact and the diagnosis may be missed on hematoxylin and eosin stained sections if the clinical rule out

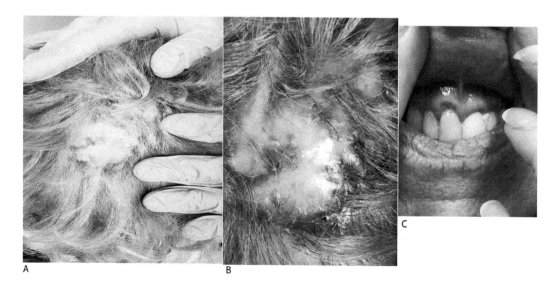

A   B   C

FIGURE 29.10 (A, B) BPCP shows scarring alopecia area with crusts on the scalp and (C) focal involvement of the gingival mucosa.

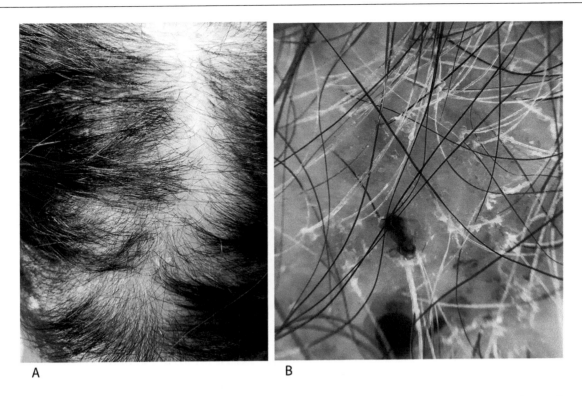

FIGURE 29.11 (A) Another subtle case of BPCP presenting with focal areas with blisters and crusts resulting in scarring alopecia. Trichoscopy shows non-specific findings of erythema and hemorrhagic crusts (B, ×20). This case has been managed for lichen planopilaris for years.

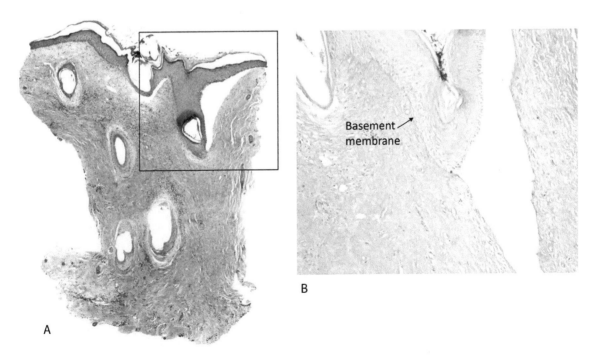

FIGURE 29.12 (A, B) There is a subepidermal cell poor cleft. At low power, this specimen could be misdiagnosed as lichen planopilaris given the similarities by the perifollicular fibrosis and lichenoid infiltrate. The cleft could be mistaken for an artifact.

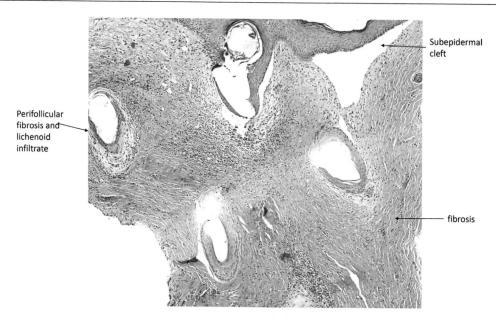

FIGURE 29.13 BPCP; note the perifollicular fibrosis and lichenoid infiltrate.

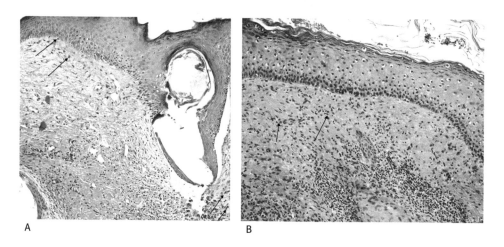

A

B

FIGURE 29.14 (A, B) Two cases of BPCP demonstrating the papillary dermal fibrosis with eosinophils in close apposition to the dermo-epidermal junction.

diagnosis does not mention BPCP; the presence of dermal fibrosis and eosinophils close to the dermo-epidermal junction should raise a concern for BPCP and direct immunofluorescence studies should be recommended in the report (Figure 29.15).

MESOTHERAPY-ASSOCIATED ALOPECIA

Mesotherapy (treatment of the mesoderm) is based on injecting vitamins, pharmaceutical and homeopathic preparations, plant extracts, vitamins, and other ingredients into the mesoderm.

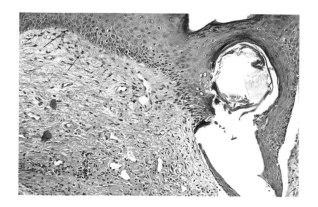

FIGURE 29.15 (A, B) A higher power view of the eosinophils in apposition to the dermo-epidermal junction, in the fibrotic stroma.

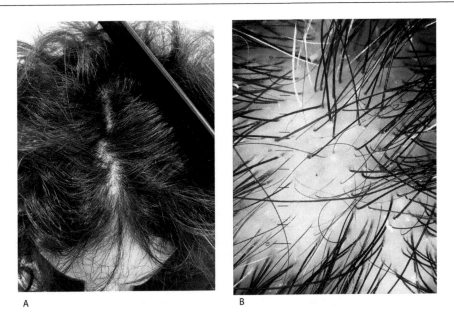

FIGURE 29.16 (A) Small patch of hair loss after mesotherapy; (B) trichoscopy shows a black dot and decreased number of terminal hairs. (Courtesy of David Saceda Corralo, MD.)

An example of mesosolution injected in the scalp would contain dutasteride, biotin and pyridoxine, among others.

- It is important to stress that the Food and Drug Administration (FDA) has not approved mesotherapy for any indication and that the Centers for Disease Control and Prevention (CDC) has recommended that "providers should inject only FDA approved products that are prepared following guidelines to ensure sterility as described in the FDA's good manufacturing practices".
- There is a lack of data regarding the efficacy and safety profile of mesotherapy for hair loss.
- Described side effects include *acute patchy alopecia* and *multifocal scalp abscess*es with subcutaneous fat necrosis and scarring alopecia (Figures 29.16 and 29.17).

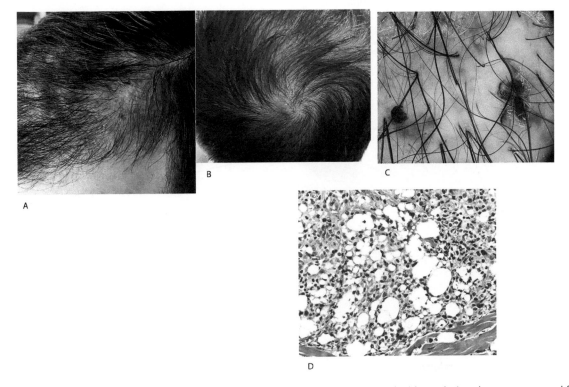

FIGURE 29.17 (A, B) Abrupt onset of inflammatory painful nodules in a patient injected with a solution that was prepared for topical drug delivery application. It contained silicone polymers. (C) Trichoscopy shows non-specific hemorrhagic crusts and erythema (×20). (D) The pathology confirms silicone granulomas. (Courtesy of Giselle Martins, MD, and Ana Leticia Boff, MD.)

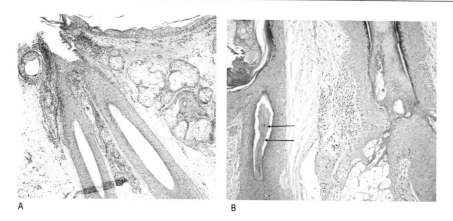

FIGURE 29.18 (A) Alopecia after mesotherapy – non-specific periinfundibular lymphocytic infiltrate without perifollicular fibrosis. The sebaceous glands are intact. (B) Note the distorted hair shaft (trichomalacia, black arrows).

- *Pathology*
  - Non-specific periinfundibular lymphocytic infiltrate that should not be mistaken for the lichenoid infiltrate in lichen planopilaris (Figure 29.18).
  - Catagen/telogen shift with trichomalacia – this pattern is indistinguishable from trichotillomania and pressure-induced alopecia and has been described also in filler induced alopecia (Figures 29.18 and 29.19).
  - It is unclear if the findings are direct effect from the injected substances leading to abrupt apoptosis and inflammation (hence, the catagen shift) or indirect effect from intravascular injection of the overfilled materials causing compression (hence, the trichomalacia), or from both.

PERMANENT ALOPECIA AFTER CHEMOTHERAPY

Permanent alopecia after chemotherapy (PAAC) is a devastating, irreversible form of hair loss, which has been mostly reported with busulfan (in patients undergoing hematopoietic stem cell transplant) and docetaxel (in patients treated for breast cancer).

- A recent study showed a trend for more severe alopecia in those receiving also an aromatase inhibitor or tamoxifen.

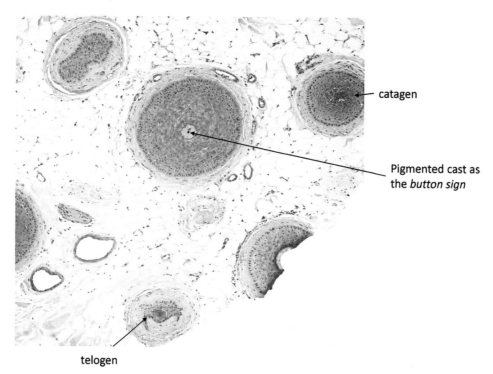

catagen

Pigmented cast as the *button sign*

telogen

FIGURE 29.19 Abrupt catagen/telogen shift with pigmented casts – this image is indistinguishable from trichotillomania or pressure-induced alopecia (and has been reported with filler-induced alopecia).

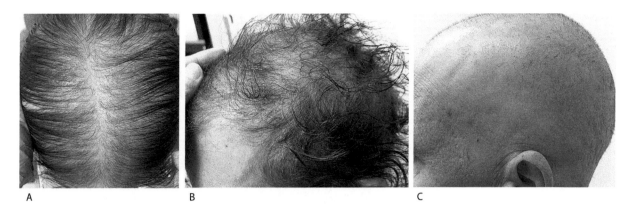

FIGURE 29.20 Permanent alopecia after chemotherapy in three women who have been treated with busulfan prior to bone marrow transplant and had normal hair in the past. The hair loss presents as (A) severely diffuse, (B) patchy and diffuse, and (C) alopecia universalis-like severely diffuse alopecia.

- The incidence of PAAC was detected as 16% among 263 children treated with busulfan prior to bone marrow transplant and 23.3% among 245 patients receiving docetaxel for breast cancer.
- Conditioning regimen with busulfan and acute Graft versus Host Disease are independent risk factors for developing PAAC.
- Most patients present with significantly reduced hair density (diffuse alopecia) of thin, sparse and short hair (complaining of hair not growing) which most choose to camouflage by wearing a wig; three clinical patterns have been described: (1) severe diffuse; (2) mostly pronounced as hair thinning on the vertex (androgen dependent area) and (3) diffuse and patchy (Figure 29.20).
- Eyebrow and eyelash alopecia is rare.
- Trichoscopy is non-specific: yellow dots, empty follicles, hair shaft variability and short regrowing hairs (Figure 29.21).
- *Pathology* is non-specific and requires clinical correlation and assessment of horizontal sections.

- Overall, a non-scarring pattern with a preserved number of follicular units; there could be areas of follicular dropout due to non-cycling fibrous streamers in the dermis but fibrotic tracts per se are usually missing (Figures 29.22 and 29.23).
- The hair counts reveal decreased number of terminal follicles, with increased telogen count and increased miniaturized vellus-like follicles with a terminal-to-vellus ratio of 1:1 (Figures 29.22 and 29.23).
- Branching strands of follicular epithelium: telogen germinal unit-like structures are noted in groups in some cases (Figure 29.24).
- There is increased number of fibrous streamers in both reticular dermis and subcutis (Figures 29.22 and 29.23).
- Reporting the follicular counts and ratios is important to the patient and the clinician as numbers in the range of 20–30 follicles per a 4 mm punch biopsy (mostly telogen germinal unit-like follicles and vellus follicles) could provide rationale for therapeutic attempt for improvement (Figure 29.25).

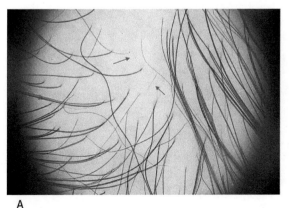

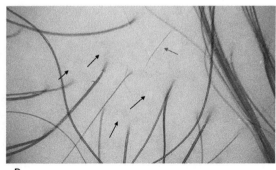

FIGURE 29.21 Empty dots (black arrow) and short regrowing hairs (red arrows) in a patient with PAAC (A, ×40; B, ×60).

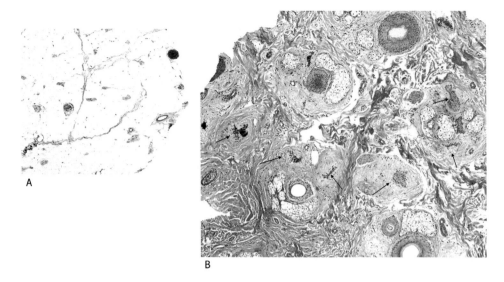

FIGURE 29.22   (A) The fat is empty with increased number of fibrous streamers. (B) There is overall preserved follicular architecture with normal sebaceous glands but most follicles are replaced by vellus follicles and telogen germinal unit-like follicular structures (arrows).

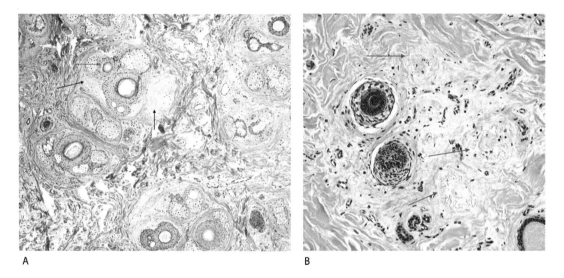

FIGURE 29.23   (A) Focal follicular dropout (black arrows), increased number of vellus follicles (red arrows) in PAAC. (B) Note the hyalinized non-cycling fibrous streamers in the dermis (red arrows).

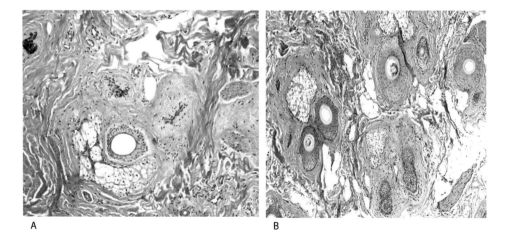

FIGURE 29.24   (A, B) Telogen germinal unit-like follicles in increased number and in groups in PAAC.

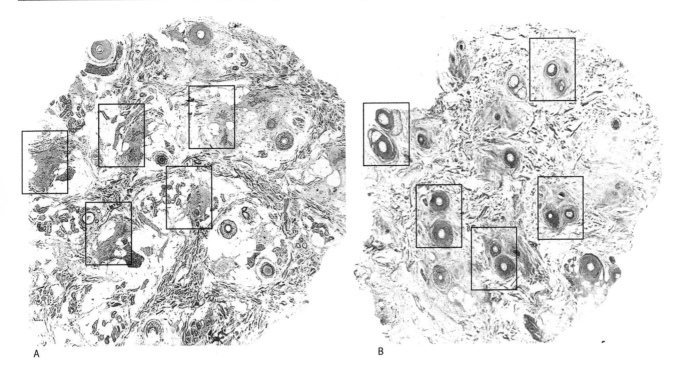

FIGURE 29.25 (A, B) Differentiation of the groups of telogen germinal unit-like follicular structures into intermediate size terminal anagen follicles is possible in some patients with a complex therapeutic regimen. (Courtesy of Giselle Martins, MD, and Anal Leticia Boff, MD.)

FURTHER READING

Bresters D, Wanders DCM, Louwerens M, Ball LM, Fiocco M, van Doorn R. Permanent diffuse alopecia after haematopoietic stem cell transplantation in childhood. Bone Marrow Transplant. Jul 2017;52(7):984–8.

Brunsting LA, Perry HO. Benign pemphigold: a report of seven cases with chronic, scarring, herpetiform plaques about the head and neck. AMA Arch Derm. 1957;75(4):489–501.

Duque-Estrada B, Vincenzi C, Misciali C, Tosti A. Alopecia secondary to mesotherapy. J Am Acad Dermatol. 2009 Oct; 61(4):707–9.

Fonia A, Cota C, Setterfield JF, Goldberg LJ, Fenton DA, Stefanato CM. Permanent alopecia in patients with breast cancer after taxane chemotherapy and adjuvant hormonal therapy: clinicopathologic findings in a cohort of 10 patients. J Am Acad Dermatol. 2017 May;76(5):948–57.

Katta R, Nelson B, Chen D, Roenigk H. Sarcoidosis of the scalp: a case series and review of the literature. J Am Acad Dermatol. 2000 Apr;42(4):690–2.

Khunkhet S, Rattananukrom T, Thanasarnaksorn W, Suchonwanit P. Alopecia induced by autologous fat injection into the temporal area: case report and review of the literature. Case Rep Dermatol. 2019 Jun 5;11(2):150–6.

La Placa M, Vincenzi C, Misciali C, Tosti A. Scalp sarcoidosis with systemic involvement. J Am Acad Dermatol. 2008;59(5 Suppl):S126–7.

Lim J, Salih Z, Tetlow C, Wong H, Thorp N. Permanent hair loss associated with taxane chemotherapy use in breast cancer: a retrospective survey at two tertiary UK cancer centres. Eur J Cancer Care (Engl). 2020 Dec 22:e13395.

Lutz ME, Pittelkow MR. Progressive generalized alopecia due to systemic amyloidosis. J Am Acad Dermatol. 2002;46(3):434–6.

Miteva M, Misciali C, Fanti PA, Vincenzi C, Romanelli P, Tosti A. Permanent alopecia after systemic chemotherapy: a clinicopathological study of 10 cases. Am J Dermatopathol. Jun 2011;33(4):345–50.

Miteva M, Wei E, Milikowski C, Tosti A. Alopecia in systemic amyloidosis: trichoscopic-pathologic correlation. Int J Trichology. 2015;7(4):176–8.

Plachouri KM, Georgiou S. Mesotherapy: safety profile and management of complications. J Cosmet Dermatol. 2019 Dec;18(6):1601–5.

Torres F, Tosti A, Misciali C, Lorenzi S. Trichoscopy as a clue to the diagnosis of scalp sarcoidosis. Int J Dermatol. 2011;50(3):358–61.

Trichoscopy in Hair Restoration Practice: An Introduction for Hair Restoration Surgeons and Pathologists[*]

30

Giselle Martins, MD, and Rui Oliveira Soares, MD

Contents

Hair restoration or hair transplant (HT) is a surgical procedure that may also be considered a form of art. It is mostly performed on the scalp as part of the management of patients with androgenetic alopecia. This chapter will focus on the use of trichoscopy in the HT. Both authors are also practicing dermatologists and have been using extensively trichoscopy to improve the outcomes of their HT patients; they share here their tips with other hair restoration surgeons and help pathologists who receive scalp biopsies from hair restoration practices better understand the HT process.

GENERAL CONCEPTS ABOUT HT

- The concept of follicular unit (FU) was introduced by Headington in 1984.
- The method that we call follicular unit transplant (FUT): obtaining an elliptical long strip of skin in the donor area, microscopic dissection of the FUs and implantation, was introduced by Bernstein in 1995.

- The follicular unit extraction (FUE) consisting in obtaining with the use of a micro-punch, of cylindrical micrografts containing each one a FU, was described in 1990 by Rassman.
- It is consensual today that both methods of extraction of FUs are useful, may be combined in some cases and should be part of the arsenal of the HT surgeon. The *main advantage of FUT* is that there is no need to shave the donor area. Other important advantage is that hair density in the donor area is not reduced. *Main advantages of FUE* are being a less invasive procedure (some patients do not want a "cut") and avoiding a linear scar in the donor area (although the trichophytic suture, described by Simon Rosenbaum in 1999, has minored this problem).
- In the following decades, the use of stem cells will probably solve the problem of hair harvesting, allowing creation of an infinite number of FUs.
- In the present, some hair surgeons claim they extract part of the follicle (vertical transaction) and leave the other part in the donor area, leading to a viable FU in both donor and receptor areas. The idea is good, but the results are not reproducible by other hair surgeons and require more scientific evidence.

---

[*] Some of the material in this chapter is also contained in the chapter by Rui Oliveira Soares on Trichoscopy in hair transplantation in Rubina Alves and Ramon Grimalt, eds, *Techniques in the Evaluation and Management of Hair Disease*, CRC Press, Boca Raton and Abingdon, 2021.

MAIN ADVANTAGES IN USING TRICHOSCOPY IN HT

- **Exclude a concomitant non-scarring alopecia such as alopecia areata**

  Unrecognized autoimmune hair loss condition can be a risk factor for the success of the HT; therefore, establishing the correct diagnosis by suspecting it on trichoscopy and confirming it on pathology can prevent complications and unfavorable results (Figure 30.1).

- **Identify undetectable (by naked eye) scarring alopecia**

  Some patients have an overlapping scarring alopecia. Failure to detect this condition, and its activity, can cause the lack of success after the HT procedure. All HT surgeons should perform trichoscopy and trichoscopy-guided biopsies to exclude subtle cases of lichen planopilaris and fibrosing alopecia in a pattern distribution among others (see also Chapter 7) (Figure 30.2).

- **Measure the quality of the donor area in the planning of the HT**

  Measuring the quality of the donor area is important because it helps the surgeon to predict the result of the procedure. The extension of the safe donor area is easily determined by the naked eye. However, other important parameters are better determined by trichoscopy (with or without a phototrichogram), which is a ubiquitous and inexpensive tool.

1. *Percentage of multi-hair FUs (2, 3, 4 hairs):* probably, the most important single characteristic that may determine a good final result. To obtain density, it is crucial to harvest a high number of multi-hair FUs, especially FU with 3 and 4 hairs. Trichoscopy is a simple and inexpensive way of determining the number of hairs of each FU per optic camp in the donor area (Figure 30.3).

2. *Hair thickness:* not as determinant for the final result as the precedent, but also important. It is easily determined with trichoscopy. Thin hair in the donor area is a common problem in women; in some cases, this may be improved with pharmacological

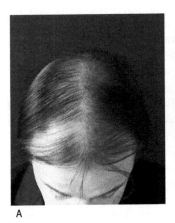 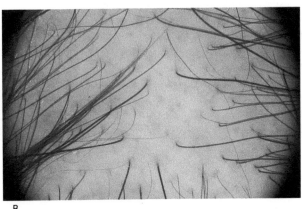

A   B

FIGURE 30.1 (A) This patient has clinically an asymmetric hair loss with patches in the androgen depended area. (B) Trichoscopy shows abrupt miniaturization and yellow dots. The diagnosis of androgenetic alopecia associated with alopecia areata was confirmed on pathology. Missing the correct diagnosis will definitely limit the results of the surgery.

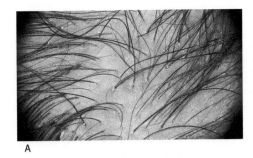 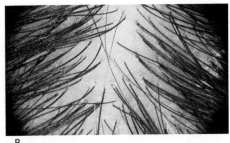

A   B

FIGURE 30.2 (A, B) Trichoscopy to exclude scarring alopecia: these patients have miniaturization of the hair shafts associated with erythema and scales. Sometimes, it could be seborrheic dermatitis associated with androgenetic alopecia but these two cases have a confirmed diagnosis on lichen planopilaris (LPP) on pathology (×40) and are therefore are not candidates for a hair transplant procedure.

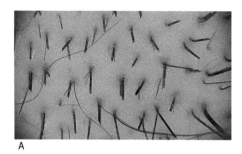
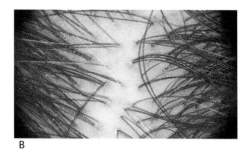

FIGURE 30.3 Trichoscopy measures the quality of the donor area: note the small number of FUs with 3 and 4 hairs in (A) and the high number of FUs in (B). The small number of FUs will definitely limit the density that is feasible to obtain with the procedure.

or non-pharmacological approaches (platelet-rich plasma, laser therapy, micro-needling, etc.).

3. *Hair density* is important because it determines the number of FUs that can be harvested per area, but also because a very low density will make more visible the FUE circular scars and the FUT linear scar. To minimize the FUE scar, a punch smaller than 0.9 mm should be used; to minimize the FUT scar, a trichophytic suture should be performed.

- **Detection of complications**
  Trichoscopy is useful for the early detection of some complications in the donor and recipient areas. Timely detection is important because immediate treatment may spare the FUs (both original and implanted).
  - *Inflammation* is a common *early complication* in the **donor area** and could be detected promptly by trichoscopy (Figure 30.4). It may be due to infection, excessive tension (in the case of FUT) or simply due to the emerging hair shafts through the skin (in case of trichophytic suture). A *late complication* is *abnormal healing* that may lead to a wide scar or, rarely, to an elevated hypertrophic scar. This may be due to incorrect technique (too much tension or lack of trichophytic suture) or to the patient's abnormal propensity for excessive scarring. In such cases,

the early detection allows a quick therapeutic intervention (with intralesional corticosteroids, for example).

- In the **recipient area**, early and long-term complications can be detected too: *Early common complications* are *crusts, folliculitis and skin inflammation*. It is important to remember that in the first 24–48 hours, the existence of micro-crusts is a normal trichoscopic finding (Figures 30.5–30.7). Big or persistent crusts may be due to poor cleaning or excessive hemorrhage and disappear in the following days. After one week, there may be *mild erythema and white vanished round areas*, probably due to the healing process. By that time, the FUs with multiple number of hairs resemble a Spanish fan, due to the big angulations between juxtaposed hairs arising from the same follicular opening (Figure 30.8). *This is a distinguishing feature of the transplanted FUs when compared with the original FUs. Long-term complications* in the recipient area are best assessed with trichoscopy (Figure 30.9): suboptimal growth (uncommon), characterized by unexpected low density, pits and cobble stoning, perifollicular elevations (considered to be due to imperfect matching the depth between the FUs and the recipient site), and unnatural hairline due to wrong distribution, direction or multi-hair FUs.

- **Assess the teamwork**
  - Trichoscopy allows to detect a high percentage of empty slits.
  - Thichoscopy may also detect FUs introduced too deep (Figure 30.10) as the implant epidermis is not seen (implant epidermis should be seen 0.5–1 mm above the surrounding skin).
  - Poor cleaning could be instantly monitored with magnification.
  - A high percentage of early uptake, most of the FUs implanted are present after few days, is a good indirect measure of good teamwork.

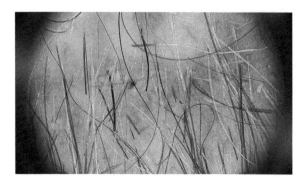

FIGURE 30.4 Inflammation in the donor area on the third day after FUT with trichophytic suture.

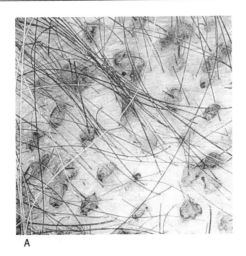
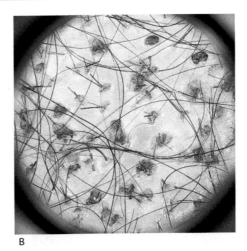

FIGURE 30.5   Normal (A) and abnormal (B) crusts 48 hours after hair transplant. Note that in (B) the crusts are bigger, irregular and pustular.

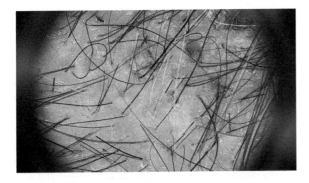

FIGURE 30.6   Many pustular lesions in a patient coming from a hair transplant in the context of "a medical holiday" in a Middle Eastern country.

- In the long term, pits and cobble stoning (perifollicular elevations) are indicative of bad teamwork, meaning bad matching between FUs and recipient sites.
- A suboptimal growth is usually not due to incorrect teamwork, but often related to a specific patient condition.
- Finally, a nice single-hair-FU irregular hairline (meaning that it will look natural) may be checked with trichoscopy.

• **Assess the effect of complementary treatments**
The surgeon may use the transplant session to perform another kind of invasive treatment in areas outside the recipient area. Platelet-rich plasma and micro-needling are good examples. In some cases, especially if the number of avoidable FUs is not high, the surgeon may concentrate the implants in

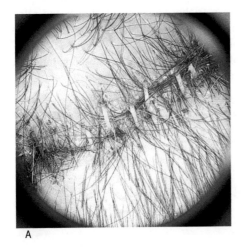
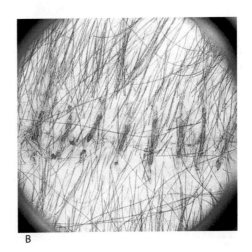

FIGURE 30.7   (A) The FUT suture in the same patient as in Figure 30.6; note that many adjacent hairs were trapped by the suture. (B) A normal aspect of a trichophytic suture by day 7 (in both cases, an absorbable suture was used).

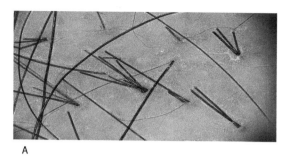
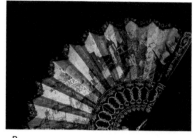

A   B

FIGURE 30.8   (A) Low-density area of implants in a woman: the implanted multi-hair FUs show big angulations between juxtaposed hairs, resembling (B) a Spanish fan.

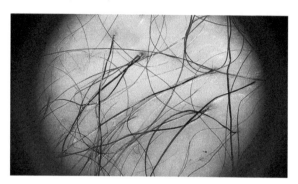

FIGURE 30.9   Perifollicular elevations (due to imperfect matching in the depth between the FUs and the recipient site) 6 months after hair transplant in a scalp scar due to craniotomy. Note the high number of dystrophic hairs, typical of FUs implanted in hypertrophic scars.

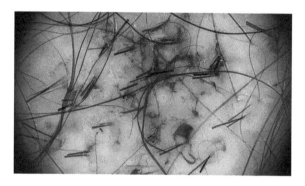

FIGURE 30.10   Trichoscopy as a tool to assess teamwork: in this image immediately after HT, most of the slits have an implant but most of the implants are placed too deep. Epidermis from each implant should be 0.5–1 mm above the scalp epidermis.

a reduced recipient area and stimulate the rest of the affected scalp. This approach is particularly useful in women. In such cases, trichoscopy is a good tool to compare before/after images of the complementary treatment in the non-implanted area (Figure 30.11). It is important to note that the natural course of the androgenetic alopecia will determine the level of thinning in the non-treated androgen-dependent area.

- **Assess the result of HT and increase the patient's compliance and the surgeon's confidence**
  Showing images proving the improvement increases patient's compliance. The classical global photography is a very good tool for this purpose; however, demonstrating what happens at a follicular level helps the patient's understanding of the improvement (Figure 30.12). It may help in explaining the limitations of the method (by showing the quality of the donor area, namely thickness, density and most importantly the percentage of FUs with more than three hairs).

In conclusion, the surgeon gets confident with the use of trichoscopy not only because they can better evaluate the results of the HT, but also because they can (1) detect subtle cases of lichen planopilaris prior to the procedure by performing a trichoscopy-guided biopsy and refer these patients for further pharmacological treatment, (2) identify complications of the HT procedure, and (3) assess the team's work. In the case of a suboptimal result, trichoscopy may be useful to detect the cause (example: the existence of cicatricial alopecia).

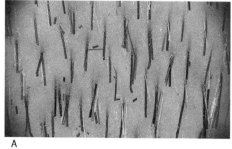
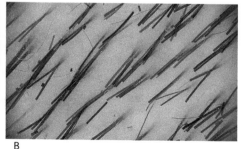

A   B

FIGURE 30.11   Trichoscopy as a tool to assess PRP treatment in a non-transplanted androgen-dependent area in the procedure (A) 1 day and (B) 3 months later. Note the increase of the number of follicular units with 3 and 4 hairs.

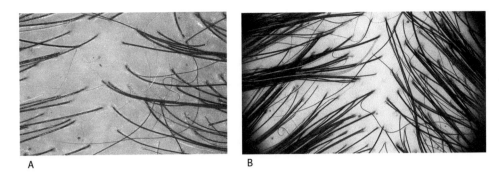

FIGURE 30.12   Trichoscopy as a tool to assess the results of the treatment in a non-transplanted androgen-dependent area (A, before; B, 12 months after). Note the increase of the number of follicular units with 3 and 4 hairs and improvement of the honeycomb network.

Index

Note: Locators in *italics* represent figures and **bold** indicate tables in the text.

*For Product Safety Concerns and Information please contact
our EU representative GPSR@taylorandfrancis.com Taylor & Francis
Verlag GmbH, Kaufingerstraße 24, 80331 München, Germany*

T - #0187 - 160425 - C220 - 280/210/10 [12] - CB - 9781138313538 - Gloss Lamination